This was written over the best part of a year when depression had me at my lowest, I lost so many friends because of the grip this debilitating and downright destructive disease had on me. I chose to write because I needed to. It wasn't easy and it still isn't.

November 2014

From the age of 18 I've suffered from depression. I've tried for years to let people into my mind and failed miserably. I've always felt that I've been different from everyone but I've never been able to define the exact reason why I've felt this way. My name is Dave Roberts, I'm 32, balding, a borderline alcoholic and a bit of an intentional misfit. I'm also quite good with random dates from my past, I don't know why. I've always been a social person, it's just my nature. In high school I wasn't popular but I wasn't bullied either, I just studied and just... got myself through it, I left Larbert High School in 1998 with decent standard grade results, bizarrely a two for German and a three for English, even from an early age I kind of thought that I wasn't like the rest. I've always been intrigued by the human mind and what goes on inside the head of the others, what people are thinking, worries, thoughts etc., I don't exactly know why, it's just something that has always interested me. I left school on 20/11/1998 and joined a recruitment place called JHP, I then started work with a company called 'Dunmore Transfab' on 30/11/1998 as what's known in the industry as an 'Office Junior'. I was a jobseeker, I was rake thin, I had lots of hair, had no experience but I had a way with people. I was paid £240 a month which to me at the time was a lot of money, I hadn't had that much money before and it was nice. I then left about six months later and got a job with a company I actually can't remember, funny that. I think it might have been 'Apex Consulting' but I can't remember, I was in charge with sending outgoing mail. (WOW!) One thing I definitely remember is my boss was this smug English guy, I can never remember his name so we'll call him 'Prick', basically because he was a total prick. Bald, awful taste in shirts and from what I recall (and to my annoyance) he smelt quite nice. I remember he called me in one day into his wee pokey, crummy office and he sat me down. Prick: Dave, how are you today? Me: I'm good Justin, how are you? Prick: I'm good thanks, I need to speak to you Me: Sure, everything ok? Prick: Actually, not quite. I've got a few concerns with how you pronounce words. Me: Oh, ok. Prick: We're going to go through some sentences and go from there Me: Sure We then spent the next 10minutes with me saying words and sentences and him writing them down with how I spoke and how he felt they should have been written,(nice eh?) I have quite a thick Scottish accent, it's not Fife thick but it's not Edinburgh thin either, I consider myself to pronounce things well in a professional environment, but in 1998 maybe I was still a little bit too raw. Anyways, I kept this list that he'd written and amazingly I thanked him at the time for 'helping me', looking back I should have taken off my tie and strangled him with I, my parents went absolutely fucking nuts when they saw this list, I thought at one point my Dad's head was going to pop clean away from his shoulders (Aye, thanks.. prick, remind me to thank you for that as well you fucking absolute wanker.) Actually still looking back he was even more of a prick than what I remember. I was lucky to work beside a gorgeous woman by the name of Ruth, she had blonde hair, iconic Jennifer Aniston style and was just really lovely, had glasses as well, she helped me a lot when I managed to make a balls up of the franking machine. One day 'Prick' came into the office with his stupid shades and awful shirts and he was in a really foul mood, I mean... an AWFUL mood, I got it first because I was the job-seeker/whipping boy. Ruth though, oh Ruth was sweet, she was one of the actual staff and was just lovely; she always smelled like coconut, I like the smell of coconut. Anyways, Prick by this point was on a warpath, in professional terms he was the equivalent of a baby throwing all toys out of his pram and poor Ruth got right in the middle of it. Looking back I now term it 'Hurricane Prick'. Ruth was REALLY upset, he made her cry and that made me really sad. Although I was only 16 I made her a cup of tea/coffee and asked I she'd like to go outside, she accepted and we went outside, Ruth accepted, had a wee bubble and then felt better so we went back in. I didn't last too long there, it didn't feel right and working for that bawbag eventually became too much for me, I sought alternative employment. My first full-time job was with TSC in Larbert, I'd went for about thirty interviews before this but just couldn't land a job. When I got the job I remember getting the letter, legging it up the stairs and shouting on my Dad who was in the toilet at the time, I remember peering under the door and saw his slippers, I now feel bad because it's now obvious to me he was having a shit. (sorry Dad, I was excited!) I now had my first professional job at the age of 18, I started on 30/11/2000 and I was a 'Customer Service Associate', shortened to CSA just for the sake of being an acronym I assume. I was so excited to get the job, I was now earning £1000 a month and would happily give my Mum £100 a month for rent. My Mum is the best person ever, she is so caring, so strong and such a rock for our family, I love both my parents very much.. I mean, I idolise my parents but I'll talk about that a little bit later.

So I started with TSC (Telecom Service Centres) on 30/11/2000, I was so proud that I'd found a job and I was now on my way in life, high school was over and now I was ready to start my working life. For the first four years it was brilliant, I met so many good people and to this day I'm still friends with, just to name a few that I'm still friends with today there's Erin Docherty, Blair Brodie, Lia Radtkowska , Lynda Simpson, Shirley Duncan, Diana Boreman and Kellie McEwan. Over the first three years I was very productive, over a 12 hour shift I would have less than one minute wrap/after call work, for those that have never worked in a call centre this is the amount of time you need to leave notes on a customers account. I was awesome, I had my nice wee shirts and ties, I was super-punctual and I just... got on with it. I was young, thin, had blue hair (which was my passport picture!) and would go to a pub called Grubowski's on a Friday, terrible pub but great jukebox and pool table, I had soooo many good times there, it's here that my love/addiction to alcohol was born. In 2003 a job offering came up, it was with Hutchison 3G (or 3 as it was known) and it was for the role of 'Retentions Adviser', 3 were the first people to roll out '3G' on mobile networks, before this the closest you got to the internet was 'WAP' (Wireless Application Protocol), mobile services had evolved from 1G (Calls) to 2G (Calls & text messages) then 2.5G (Calls, texts and MMS/picture messages) to 3G. (Calls, texts, MMS/Picture messages and videos/internet connectivity) I was lucky enough to get the job and in 2003 I started in 3 whilst being a part of TSC, we got a bus from Larbert to Glasgow everyday and the shifts were between 8:30am – 4:30pm and 10:30am to 6:30pm (I think?) and we got a bus back to TSC at the end of the shift. The job itself was ok, I couldn't realise offer anything for customers to cancel as at the time I believe 3 had around 40% network coverage across the UK and they had two phones, the NEC 606 (big) and an NEC 808. (Clamshell, shaped, HUGE! I remember recording my Dad at the golf course with it and I think the video quality was about 144p, grainy/awful. You could download Barclays Premier League goals as they went in though, it was so cool being able to look at goals going in, being a huge Liverpool fan though it was very rare I actually got to see any of their goals) 3 had a really good culture, it was casual dress and we were there with TSC Greenock, to this day I've got a few friends from there, I've not been as good a friend to these people as I should have, for this I apologise. At the time the customer could either pay their Early Termination Fee or we could offer something like £10 off, I 'retained' a lot of customers that way, in fairness, it wasn't really a retention, not a lot of people had that money to cancel a contract, I certainly didn't! I really liked

3 and it was a place I thought I may look at in the future. The culture was relaxed yet professional and the fact that it was casual dress just made me like the place even more My Dad's name is Davy and my Mum's name is Nancy, my Dad is now 67 years old and my Mum is 65 years old. I have two brothers, Chris who is 45, is married to his wife Morven and have two beautiful kids named Scott and Katie. I stay with my brother Steve, he's like a silent rock for me but I've never been able to tell him this. We just have a really good time together, we're always making each other laugh and we just talk utter crap, it's brilliant! I apologise to Chris and Morven, although I'm an Uncle to Scott and Katie I've never been there for them, partly due to my fear of children, mostly due to the fact I can't go longer than two minutes without swearing, I swear a lot, an awful fucking lot, it gets me in trouble sometimes as I've got a HUGE booming voice which I swear can be heard for miles. Remember 'The Jungle Book' where Mowgli gets in trouble and Baloo shouts 'BAGHHEEERRAAA! BAAGGGHHERAAAAA' and he's right there? That's what I'm like, I have a huge voice, to be honest I'm not sure whether this is a good thing or a bad thing. I know a lot of people will say the same thing but I'm really protective of my family, they are the people in my life that mean the most to me, they always have and they always will. Growing up I always

remember Davy would go up the town on a Saturday, he would go up to just have a browse around Falkirk and me and Steve would normally go with him. He'd look at books, shirts, everything really, he was a pro at browsing, he still is. Me & Steve had a Sega Mega Drive at the time (SEEEGGGA!) and he would get fleeced every time for a game, the main ones he got tucked up with were PGA Tour Golf II, Micro Machines and Pete Sampras Tennis, actually PGA Tour Golf II still has the Woolworths sticker on it with a price tag of £39.99, looking back it's amazing to think that at the time this was the most graphically up-to-date and playable game, I still play it and I'm happy to admit it. I still have my Mega Drive and I can frequently still be seen playing Road Rash I & II (Damn you Helldog, I hate you so much.. you always knock me off my bike you big fat fucker. I actually remember Road Rash II, there was this butch woman named 'Public Enemy No. 1', (original eh?) I won a race and there would be a little caption at the end, 9 times out of 10 it would be sour grapes by the person that was second, I always remember that Public Enemy No. 1 said 'I like to douse the winner in Petrol and set them on Fire, not that I'm jealous'.. I mean, I know it's a street race but does anyone else find that a little bit harsh? I was a ten year old boy playing a game in our box room and she's coming out with things like that. Makes me glad that I always whooped her. I took great pleasure in over-taking her, slowing down and then just knocking off her bike. Take that, cow. To this day I'm still thankful for my upbringing by my parents, I got away with absolutely nothing and when I did something out of line my Mum smacked my arse so hard, it went babboon red and would glow for hours, I was afraid of her, I still am! My Mum is also big on Sunday names so me, Steve and Chris are actually called David, Steven & Christopher, I respect that about my Mum, we're always going to be her little boys and I'm fine with her calling me this. The only other person that gets away with calling me David is Claire Fullerton, I love her a lot and she's been my best friend for years, she's gorgeous, amazing and has always been there for me. (Thank you dear x)) The thing I liked most about my childhood was that at the end of the school term we'd go away for a week, my fave time was when we went to Leven up in 'The Kingdom of Fife', it's the one I remember the most, partly because it was the only time that I've seen a seal but mostly because I couldn't understand why the sea would be further away when I woke up than it was when I went to my bed, I swore the caravan had moved in the middle of the night, as I was to later discover, it was infact the tide. What a tit I was. My family are amazing though, they've been there for me when I've done some pretty stupid things, the fact they've continually forgiven me humbles me so much, I could not ask for better parents. I've always felt I've been different from people, it's just a feeling that I've had since I turned 17/18 and it's something I've never been able to shift. I've always had a phrase going through my head and I've just never been able to decrypt it, here it is: 'I've always felt my mind was right for my body, I was just born at the wrong time'. I can't tell you just why this started but it's just always been there, eternally circling the back of my mind before making a dash to the front, then back again, during my depression periods it just sits there on it's wee perch at the front of my mind, singing the line to me over and over again. Actually, at my worst times of suffering (2011 and now) my head feels like a fireworks display that doesn't end or a vortex that continually swirls for days at a time, I have so many thoughts and I just can't grasp one, it causes my vision of myself to distort and it causes me no end of problems communicating with anyone. I'll be frank, I have tried for so many years to keep people out, I struggle with letting people in and to be honest I've never wanted to let anyone in. It would be false for me to say I like being depressed but I do find positives in it, for example I find when I'm at work my productivity and call quality go up as I'm physically unable to talk to anyone, my mind shuts down but runs in a sort of 'safe mode' so I can function day-to-day in my work, it's a surreal period when it happens, I'd love to let you in and just see what I'm seeing and feel what I'm feeling, it's truly terrifying the thoughts I manage daily, you probably wouldn't believe it. I don't think I give myself enough credit, I never have. I find it easier to criticise myself and rip into things I don't think I've done perfectly, I set myself stupidly high standards, I always have and that just doesn't help. My relationship with alcohol is a bad one, if it was a relationship status on Facebook it would be 'It's Complicated', I've been a borderline alcoholic for the best part of 10years, I always thought I was in control of my drinking but during this period I've been reflecting and alcohol has definitely controlled me. It's been one of the causes of my current fight with depression, I saw it happening yet I chose to do nothing about it, I ignored it and here I am, off work and seeing doctors, clinical psychiatrists and in the near future I may even have to see a psychologist. I think about death a lot, I have an unhealthy obsession with it and I always have done. I've pictured my funeral a lot and the song I would have to send me off to be burnt to ashes, it's a tossup between a song by 'Rise Against' called 'Elective Amnesia, a song called 'This Is Not For You' by Blood Red Shoes' or 'Bullet In The Head' by the legendary 'Rage Against The Machine'. At my funeral I wouldn't have people mourning, I'd have all sorts of bright colours and wigs, air horns and funny noises because I don't believe death should be mourned, it should be life being celebrated. Besides, I wouldn't want people crying over me, I'll miss people one thousand times more than they could ever miss me. I find it strange that I'm saying this because suicide is such a selfish act, from the age of 18 I've never really seen myself past the age of 35, it's just something I've always felt and to be honest I still feel that way, I don't envisage myself making it past that age, I don't see myself getting old like my Dad and having a few pints in my local, I never have seen myself getting to that . To be honest I'm not 100% sure that I'm going to make it through this... I've always thought of myself as one of the good guys, a nice guy, a popular guy. To be 100% honest I don't think that I give myself enough credit at times, I am very hard on myself, mainly because I set myself very high standards and this isn't the first time that my mind has short-circuited. When I was 20 and working at TSC, I was lucky enough to make some really good friends, friends that appreciated who I was and friends that I still think about regularly. I over-think, if overthinking was a profession I could see me being Chief Operating Officer, my mind never stops thinking, I liken it to a PC that's not turned off/idle. Although it's not doing anything there's still processes going and things taking up space. I've always viewed myself as someone who just.. never fit in, an outcast, a third wheel and the like. I've always secretly resented people who were super-popular, people who had a knack of just being funny and good -looking guys who always managed to bed a different woman every Friday & Saturday night. Actually, thinking of it I really don't like many people, thinking of my day-to-day life I shout a lot at the endless amount of crap, monotonous adverts that are on TV, I shout at the TV during the football and even when I'm playing the Mega Drive I do the same. Good god, I'm so angry at everything and I hate people, no wonder I'm single. Actually, that's a whole other topic, I'll try to touch on it later and keep it brief. (Unlikely) So, friends & family, the people on this earth that mean the most to me , if it wasn't for them I would actually be dead by now, well.. there is one friend that is special to me, and when I say 'special' I mean I have a special relationship with him. I don't think it's fair to mention his name but all I'll say is he drives me 'Pottie'. I first met this roving scallywag in 2006, I'd just started working at 3 and was getting on ok. Unfortunately the job I was doing was shipped and I got offered the chance to join another department. I accepted and in March 2007 I turned up for my first day, I lasted half a day, went to the pub and got drunk, talk about getting off to a flier! To this day I don't know what caused me to do it, I often re-visit this day and just can't fathom what was going through my head. Unfortunately this wasn't an isolated incident, I have several events in my life that I frequently re-visit and pour over again and again, I made a lot of mistakes, I make a lot of mistakes. So this chap 'Pottie', he started off ok, he sat with his headphones in a lot and was a wee bit deaf, well... the fact that you had to shout on him to get attention was an indication that he was in-fact, deif as a post. It was a good time, I was enjoying my job and just life in general, I was 24, earning a decent wage and I was beginning to establish myself amongst society. (or so I thought) I got to know this lad very well and to this day we're still friends/friendly enemies. I'm quite an easy guy to wind-up, actually I'm one of the easiest guys to wind up, I'm also quite gullible so I fall for things I perhaps I shouldn't. Sometimes it's all an act and I just do it for the attention, I'd be flat out lying if I said otherwise. Anyways, I digress... this guy means the world to me and I do actually care for him, it's just, he sometimes gets on my tits, I'm pretty sure I get on his too at points. The thing about him is that he is a naturally funny guy and the fact he has a richt' thick Fifer accent adds to the comedy. I'll start with the negatives about him and I'm 99.9% certain I've said the majority of these things to him on one of my many tirades at him during our tumultuous, strange and sometimes (emotionally) violent relationship. He is a sleekit, beady-eyed, crafty, mop-haired, manipulative arsehole who has given me such reprehensible nick-names like 'Bambo', 'Rambunctious Roberts' and often refers to my hometown as 'Hallglen', I don't stay in Hallglen, I've never stayed in Hallglen and I don't have any intentions of staying in Hallglen. He always makes jokes about my dear old Mum, on many a night out I've made the casual threat of killing him, he understands this though. I've got various drawings of me by him, I'll start by saying he is quite the artist, he is also a damn good piss-artist. I can't actually remember how it started but at one point I had around 12 drawings depicting me in various precarious positions. The drawings follow a few set templates, I always have a light-bulb shaped head for example, I've always got an NHS plaster on my forehead , I can only assume that's where the dick has been removed from my forehead. (Cunt) My dog Cassie died in April this year, she was 13 and a half and I loved her to bits, by the end she really had no control over her body and one of her final acts was to spray projectile shit over a nice new pair of white trainers I'd bought, god bless her the wee lamb. (I miss you dear) I left 3 in May 2014 to explore new adventures, before I went I got a nice wee card from my friends and of course the obligatory drawing by the man affectionately named 'Mr P'. It had highlighted various events that I'd been involved in at 3 but the part of the drawing that I want to draw attention to was a sign, it wasn't the most prominent part of the drawing, bear in mind I left 3 two weeks after the death of my wee lifelong pal. The sign that got my attention stated 'Hell: 5 Miles, (Cassie's there)', now if anyone else had the audacity/balls to even mention Cassie in a derogatory manner I would rip the head clean off their shoulders, find some rugby posts and then proceed to punt their head over them. This shows how good a relationship I actually had with him because not only did I not kill him, I burst out laughing. (Love you Mr P!) I've been really lucky with the people in my life because 98% of them have been absolutely rock solid, I'm still in contact with a lot of people from as far back as high school. I consider myself a really lucky guy in the fact I've always been able to retain friends, even when I've hit the self-destruct button and decided to just be a total arsehole to them, I thank my lucky stars that I still have them because it's not been a one-off that I've self-imploded , it's happened a lot of times so to all of you that are by my side I thank you, I sincerely and genuinely thank you. Having so many great people in my life makes the thought of suicide that much harder, suicide is something that I think regularly about, it always has been and over the past few weeks it's something that I'm thinking of more and more. If I don't make it through this particular episode of depression I will find it pretty hard to say goodbye to those I care most about, at the same time though I am in a tremendous amount of pain and it's hard for me to keep the fight up, it is such an energy-sapping process and some days it just leaves me so drained and devoid of any fight, some days I do come close to giving up and I look at ways that I can end my life, I'm not ashamed to admit this as it's something that I regularly contemplate. I make no apologies for this and I do believe that one day that I will end my own life, either when my parents pass away or the pressures and pain become too much. I wouldn't say I've accepted that I'll take my own life, I would say that my friends and family will need to accept it. I don't know why I started writing all of this, I don't know if it was for my own benefit, if it was a last entry before I take my own life or simply it was to try and let other people in to what goes through my mind on a daily basis. I genuinely feel that there is still a stigma associated with mental health issues, personally I feel like it's a frowned upon illness and not treated with the respect and attention that it deserves. I've been quite lucky in my life because my friends have always respected the fact that I had occasional bad days and that I just couldn't talk to them, I've always respected that and to my friends that know of my suffering I really appreciate your support and your understanding, it really means a lot to me. I have never been able to talk to my friends openly about my suicidal feelings, in fact the first time I openly talked about it was on 16/10/2014 with my GP and that was only because I felt he had the right to know that I was seriously contemplating suicide, I still am but now I've got it out in the open I don't feel like I'm carrying it on my own, I have an amazing support network around me and now I've got it out in the open it doesn't feel as bad as it once did. As I said earlier though I don't think I'll be able to discuss this openly with them though, I just don't think that I could do that to friends or family. If I don't make it through this and I do take my own life I would like to apologise to everyone around me for quitting, at this specific point in time (16/10/2014 – 30/10/2014) I'm not confident I will get through the other side, I've been suffering for way too long and the fact I've got such a low opinion of myself steers me towards the possibility of suicide. I pray that I prove myself wrong, I really hope I do and live a long and prosperous life, I hope to see myself in my 60's & 70's and passing away when the reaper calls time on my existence. Although I try really hard to picture it, I just can't. I'll close this chapter with another phrase that goes through my head often. I always liken it to walking down a street, if you're always looking backwards then you're never going to get to where you're intending. "You can't see where you're going if you're always looking back"

I'm a selfless person and a selfish person. I'm selfless in the fact that I'm very accommodating, in work I'll always do things like shift swaps, overtime and staying on late if call queues, I'll bend over backwards for my family and friends and generally speaking I'm a flexible, giving person. Well, that's what people see in my day-today life, the harsh truth that people don't realise is I am actually a very, very selfish person. I'm a total pro at cancelling plans with people, I do things solely on my own priorities and generally speaking I'm a bit of an arse to people, I've tried to figure it out but I just can't. All I know is I like being on my own more than I like being in the company of others. I touched on earlier how I feel that I am different from other people, I never stop thinking about this, it is always at the forefront of my thoughts, I can't even make a simple cup of coffee without over-thinking, I always wonder how I could have made this cup better, when I'm doing my ironing I'm never satisfied with the final product, I doubt every single thing I do, I can't switch off, the light is always on, the machine always whirs, I always curse myself, I always hate myself. The fact that I have actually come to terms with my own death in itself is a very selfish thing. I'm currently sitting at my parents house (31/10/2014) gladly typing this as my folks sit less than six feet away from me, I'll have a laugh with my brother all the while thinking about suicide. It used to hurt, I mean it used to make me ache, it made me upset and would cause me to cry. The fact that this is no longer happening means that I've come to terms with the fact it's how my life will end, the thing that really gets me though is after I'm gone it'll leave such a hole, I am a good guy. I'm patient, attentive, warm, friendly, tolerant, open-minded and non-judgmental. I refuse to get drawn into arguments on social media. (God the one on Scottish Independence nearly finished me off on Facebook, I came so close so many times to telling people just to cram it. Seriously friends fell out over a debate, I'm all for opinions but not ones that get crammed right down your throat whilst not being able to g et your own point across. I hated the independence debate on social media, it really pissed... me...off) It's something I've never really got to be honest, arguing. An argument never stays on topic, it can start with something as trivial as not shutting the fridge door correctly and within ten minutes you're bringing stuff up that happened three months ago or calling the person you're arguing with something personal like an arsehole or a cunt,

I mean... this started off with something trivial like a fridge door or a light being left on and now it's like an episode of Jerry Springer. 'This Week On Jerry Springer: My cunt of a boyfriend is an arsehole, he left the fridge door open and now I hate him'. What does arguing actually resolve? All that happens is it gets out of control, people get hurt and inevitably something gets said that just... cannot be taken back. I've always been intrigued by the human mind, it's just something that interests me. I think a lot about all of it's processes, like all of the things that you remember from years and years ago. I'll give you an example. My brain still remembers an episode of 'Hey Arnold', Arnold's best friend Gerald gets tonsillitis, he's supposed to sing in some school play but it causes his voice to go all broken and high-pitched, I remember he's singing with Arnold on the bridge and a kid goes past on a bridge and says (in a crazy voice) "Hahahahaha what a crazy voice'. I remember that but on a daily basis I can forget numbers for important callbacks, mobile phones, taking the rubbish out but yet I remember episodes of Rugrats, I remember all of the kids names, Tommy, Chucky, Phil, Lil and Angelica, Tommy's Dad was called Stu Pickles. I mean, I remember this, stuff that serves me no use in everyday life. I remember as a kid my friends house caught fire and he had to stay with us, I farted and blew a hole in a pair of red and white pants I had, I was topless, I REMEMBER THIS! I just... remember! I'm also phenomenally good with dates, for example I left high school on 20/11/1998, I started my first job on 30/11/1998, I passed my driving test on 17/02/2003, I started with 3 on 07/11/2005. I just, get it with dates, I remember dates like I should remember everyday things. Things like that just blow my mind, I'm in love with the human mind, kind of ironic because most of the time I'm actually out of mines. I know no-one can beat death, it's the one certainty that there is in life, someday you will die, it's fact. I feel so ungrateful when I think of my suicide, I think about my upbringing, how much my parents sacrificed to give me nice things at Christmas, how they always ensured I had proper clothes for school and how they always provided a good home. I feel ungrateful when I think of everyone who has invested time in me and it could actually be all for nothing. I don't mean to leave a hole behind, I know that my death would, I'm a popular, up for a laugh guy, I'm affable, quite possibly the easiest person to get on with . You must be a first-class nobhead for me to actually dislike you, seriously. You must have a giant dick sprouting right in the middle of your forehead for me to not get on with you, I'm actually pretty easy going. (My friends would disagree, reason being the time I spend with them in pubs in Glasgow I shout all of the time, it's an act though, I'm an attention junkie, I fucking love it) One thing I would actually say that I hate are plastic people, people on the likes of Jersey/Geordie Shore for example, people that just have nothing underneath that plastic/cheap exterior. All they have are looks and are famous because of their antics on screen. How do people buy into it, I watched five minutes of Geordie Shore (wey-aye man!) and it was the most desperate, attention-seeking show I've watched. Some plastic pam was getting it on with this muscle bound meathead, it's like a 'noughties' televised Barbie & Ken, seriously, absolute pish but yet I see z-list celebrities releasing books at twenty-six called 'My Life'. I'm sorry, what? You're twenty-fucking-six, you've been in some poorly produced fucking show and you get your 'thrupney bits' out on national TV, fucking big deal, I could do that, I could rock up to one of those clubs and just whip my dinger out, would it get me lots of money? Would it make me a star, of course it fucking wouldn't , I'd get nicked by the Police for being D&D (Drunk & Disorderly) and chucked in the cells (quite rightly) for the night and then hit with an £80 fine. People used to get famous for at least doing something. I mean Milli Vanilli, god bless their souls at least pretended they could sing. Robson & Jerome went from Soldier Soldier to at least release some cringey mum-friendly pop 'music'. (I am well aware that

Jerome Flynn now appears on Game of Thrones) I don't mind people being famous for doing things, I mean as much as I think Keith Lemon is just not funny I can see why people find him funny, I just hate the culture that we are in of people being made famous for not having any discernible talent. Ok so I know that deviated from what this is about, so much goes on in my mind though and stuff like the above really gets on my tits. I'm trying so hard to reach out and get to the root of my depression, I'm searching, praying, trying desperately to find an outlet where I can finally get rid of this bile that is inside me. I actually feel like I have multiple different sides, I can't ever seem to think clearly, I hit the panic button too easily, I can't relax and I'm extremely insecure. I am trying to be as honest as possible in an attempt to open up, it's just really hard getting everything that's in my head out. I'm in the fortunate/unfortunate position of being able to see everything in my head, although I can see it it's almost like it's scrambled when I try to release it. I'm unsure of what's going to come out if I'm being 100% truthful, I just.... I just want to get rid of this, I've been off work for over two months now and it's still uncertain of when I'll be back, it's even a question of IF I'll be back, suicide is still at the forefront of my mind and until I can push that back then my fight continues. I know I've mentioned it before but I am actually a really good guy, I do a lot right but it's like my mind is stopping me from being the man I'm supposed to be. I'm a mess, I'm not sleeping, my personal hygiene is awful and I'm finding it more and more comfortable being away from people, I've still got awareness and I know this isn't good, I just.... I want to let everyone in, I genuinely do. If I was an inventor I'd invent a device that allowed you to see inside my mind. It'd be something like a tourist attraction but you'd definitely have to be eighteen or over to enter, if it was a film it'd be a horror but with some light hearted moments. Does that make sense? What I'm trying to get across by writing this is that I'm not wired in the same way as everyone else, I genuinely believe that I'm different and what I'm experiencing is a part of that feeling. Today is the third of November 2014, I'm sitting in my bedroom with the curtains drawn, the sun is poking in through a little gap in the curtains, I feel like they should be open, normality dictates when you get up in the morning you get yourself out of bed, get dressed, make your bed and then open the curtains. I've always had a sort of hatred for the light, I like the dark nights, I like the cold nights. I'm not sure if this is linked to my insecurity but I like the dark. I like the feeling of being in bed and it's pitch-black outside, I like when it's windy outside, I like when it's rainy outside. I daydream a lot and I look at the sky a lot, I'm inquisitive, I look at cloud patterns, people in their cars, people doing grocery shopping and I wonder what they're thinking, what's going on in their life, what troubles do they have , are they ok and the like. To look at me I look like any other normal thirty-two year old man, I dress nicely, I like colour co-ordinating my clothes, I like shaving my head with a razor, the feeling is immense. If this is sounding like my life is one big struggle then I apologise, it's not. 90% of the time I am a very productive, hardworking social butterfly. I'm constantly on Facebook posting random pictures, statuses and generally having good banter with my nearest and dearest, it's fun. I have a thick skin, I take a lot of abuse but it's good natured abuse, I like banter and I like giving as good as get. The other 10% of the time though... wow. I know it's tremendously clichéd but the walls close in, they really do. I feel it coming, it's like a male, mental version of the female menstrual cycle, I know it's coming, there are multiple warning signs and when I choose to either ignore them or meet them head-on my mind just capitulates, I mean it just breaks down and I can't talk to anyone. I've been battling this for the best part of fifteen years, fifteen years is nearly half of my life and it really is a battle. This is the longest amount of time that I've been away from everyone though. I've been away from people for two months and although I say to them that I miss them terribly, I don't. I'm ashamed to actually admit that but how do you tell your closest friends that you're accepting suicide, you're accepting the fact that you're giving in. You're openly saying to everyone in your life that you're quitting. That in itself is a very selfish attitude but does it bother me? Does it upset me? No. It used to, there was a time when the thought of suicide would cause me to burst into tears, I would then put in a bit of extra effort, get better and be my normal self. This time though, suicide enters my mind as frequently as what I'm having for dinner does. Even doing a simple thing like running a bath I can think of how much bubble bath to put in, water temperature, suicide, level of water I want to run etc. So you see, this time it's very different because I don't fear it now. I should be reeling from even thinking this but I don't. The only person I've been able to talk to this about openly is my GP, it helps, I mean it really helps but it doesn't mean my attitude towards it changes. It just sits there in the front of my mind, I've tried pushing it back and it just finds a way to gallop to the front again. Can you see that I'm trying to get this out? I'm giving this my all to let everyone in, friends, family, strangers. No-one should suffer like I suffer and that is in no way me being melodramatic, I am suffering really badly just now and I can't talk about it. Suicide carries a stigma with it and although it's something that I regularly think about I know what people's reaction would be if I started talking about it openly, my biggest fear was being sectioned in a hospital because I felt that people would view me as insane, to be honest I think I am, I don't think like a normal person, infact I can't even let you see these thoughts, they are way too dark for the written word, I scare myself with what I think, this is why I have to be as open as possible, get through this and then work on the other thoughts. I'm just so confused right now because I'm right in the middle of wanting to beat this and accepting that maybe I don't want to beat this. I'm rooting for option one, I really am, I have a lot to offer people and they see the good in me. The part that they don't see is what you see above. I'm trying though, god I'm trying. It almost feels like I'm trying to feel my way about this, like a boxer sizes up their opponent or a detective sizes up a suspect in an interview. I know what I feel in my head and I want it out, I want to go back to being me, I want to be free of all of this, live my life and then die. Personally I don't think that's too much to ask, I just.... I just want to get to the bottom of this and get it out not only for me to see but for other people. Other people who like me are intrigued by the fragility of the human mind, I need to let people in to this, it's became obvious that I can't deal with this alone and the only way I can see myself having a chance is to make it public. I've tried various different forms of therapy, I've tried computer based therapy courses, counselling, songwriting, poetry, even doing extreme things like isolating myself and forcing myself to miss people, I've tried surrounding myself with people and it just does...not... work. I need something to change, it's now 04/11/2014 , it's dark outside and I'm in my favourite place, bed with the curtains drawn and a really low-light. I've currently got Linkin Park playing and generally all is going well today. Today has been a really good day, I don't know if that's down to the fact I have to see my GP tomorrow and I'm keen to show him that I'm improving. I don't know if it's because I've not had a drink in 65 days, I don't know if it's maybe just a good couple of days that I'm having. One thing I do know though and it's that suicide is still in my head, it's still just... there and I can't seem to move it. It's a very strange state of affairs and it's a weird feeling, it's like I'm happy but with a kind of nervous energy, I'm not just happy it's like a hybrid of anxiety and happiness, I suppose I could just call it 'anxietness' or 'happexity'. Well, I feel happexity. I'm content with that feeling and I'm keen to see where it's going to take me, I hope that it takes me somewhere good.

This is beginning to feel like I'm going down a rabbit hole, going into the unknown, the unexpected and unsure of what's going to bite me. It's a little un-nerving but at the same time I'm also a little curious about what comes out of it. Since I've started writing this one thing has became abundantly clear, I think about suicide a lot more than what I should. One of the main reasons it makes me feel awful is because I know there a lot of people in the world that are a hell of a lot worse than me, people that are fighting cancer, soldiers wounded, homeless people, victims of child abuse and domestic abuse. I've got it pretty sweet as I've had it all from the start. As I eluded to earlier I had a normal childhood, I suffered no abuse, I wasn't beaten, I didn't struggle to fit in at high school, if you look at it you would ask why I feel the way I do. I don't know why, what I would love to do is go back to the first time this actually happened and what I was thinking. What had I seen or felt that caused me to clam up and just... hide away, why did this start happening? Did I experience something that caused my feelings to heighten or did I just get to a point where I started struggling? It's still 04/11/2015, the time is 19:23 and as I write I'm currently thinking about suicide, I have anti-depressants and I could quite easily over-dose, I could just... wait for my brother to go to bed and then just.. throw myself off of the balcony, I easily could, this is how hard I am fighting against this, this is where my mind regularly goes and each time it comes I've got to fight it off. So yes there are people worse off than me, yes there are lots of people with broken homes, abuse and drugs but what I feel is real to me. It tears at everything I do, I don't even say a sentence without analysing it, thinking about wordchoice, grammar, punctuation, tone and emphasis, every single thing I say gets analysed, that's not healthy, it can't be. My mind has a lot of flaws, it feels like an operating system that you would use on a computer. The general build is sound, it's reliable and works. It's just... so full of bugs, it crashes a lot and a lot of the time it runs in a 'safemode'. When this happens it basically means I can function but there's no access to any programs, software etc. I just go to work, do my work, don't say a word to anyone and then go home. I can go days without speaking to anyone and it's not because I don't want to, I physically can't. I can go months at a time and my life is great, I'm out with my friends, I'm out in a pub every Friday with my friends celebrating the end of a working week. I'm functioning, I'm working well, I'm productive, I'm chatty and I'm just an all round happy chappie. And then... it starts, I know the signs. A few weeks before it fully starts I am almost hyper-active, I'm just confident, (I'm not a confident person..) I'll start making lots of plans with friends and I'll be super happy.

Then, I'll notice I don't quite have the same zip about myself, I'll start becoming jealous of people, I'll be drinking four, maybe five times a week, I'll find myself just going home as 'I'm just not in the mood' or 'I'm tired', lastly I'll be in the house and Kelly Clarkson "Because of You" will get played, THAT, is when I know I'm not right again. It's cyclic, it always has been and now I just deal with it as if I would a cold, I know I'll be unwell for a few days and then I'll bounce back., I'm normally down for about two or three days, I'll then pick up and then it's just business as usual. The strangest thing about the two or three days that I'm down is that although the social side of my life disappears, my work and diet improve, I'll find myself just sitting working all day without missing a beat and my appetite goes down, that's not a bad thing because I eat like a pig sometimes. (oink) I fantasise a lot, I mean a LOT and I don't mean in the good sexual way, I mean I fantasise about wrong things, it's not normal, it can't be normal for a human mind to think the things I do. I fantasise about my own death, songs I'd have , (as mentioned earlier) I think about if my parents were to die what it would be like at their funeral(s), I fantasise about singing a really emotional song on karaoke with my friends, shortly after a death to show 'how strong I am', something like 'Gone Away' by 'The Offspring' or 'I Drove All Night' by 'Roy Orbison', I always envisage myself just about holding it together and getting a big hug from all of my friends because I'm 'so brave'. It's not normal, it just... cannot be normal, personally I think I'm an insane mind trapped in a sane man's body. As I'm seeing my GP weekly I tell him everything I feel throughout the week, I mean it's totally no-holds barred, things like which days I thought of suicide, which days were good, sleeping patterns, hunger levels etc. What I cannot tell him is the thoughts I have and the thoughts I stave off daily, I really don't give myself enough credit for how strong a person I am mentally and the type of battles I win daily, I win a lot of battles, I always have but they fall in the 90% of the time that I'm... normal, in the times where I'm the 10% this is when it gets exhausting, not only do I have my cycle to contend with but I also have these thoughts to contend with. It leaves me drained, sleepy, irritable, I don't eat, I don't wash and I generally just.. sleep or lay on the couch until such times as I need to use the toilet or I get hungry and I need to eat. The picture I'm trying to paint is not that I'm some psycho who should be sectioned in a hospital or that I should be mollycoddled and given lots of sympathy. This is my life, daily my brain processes so much and sometimes it just... fails, it overloads, it falls apart. I mean considering all I think about daily I think it does a fucking good job of keeping up. It has to digest and process a lot of information, if it was a computer I would say that it's low on memory and needs to free up some space, I would recommend a good clear out, de-fragmentation of the hard drive and archived/temporary files deleting. It actually feels like a PC/laptop that was once new but just hasn't been maintained, I mean for those with a PC/laptop you know what happens, malware/adware/viruses are all common place. That's about the most accurate I can describe the inner mechanics of my mind, it's odd though because as I can see them all and I thought that it would be easy for me to get them all out, it's not, it's really not! One of my many flaws (and there are a few to be fair) is that I'm too much of a nice guy, I'm accomodating, I'm considerate, I'll deliberately stand down from an argument as I don't want to fall out with someone, basically I'm a fucking coward, I need to grow a set of balls and just man the fuck up, honestly, if you were to meet me and we started having a discussion I would wimp out, unless I know you and I'm comfortable/drunk then I'll give as good as I get, I've had some proper good debates when drunk, don't get me wrong I can't recall them as I was fucking pissed but I stand my ground, just wish I had some examples. The point being is this, for a 32 year old man I should be better than what I am, I am way too nice too people, I let them talk over me and worst of all I apologise for EVERYTHING. I mean it must get on people's tits when I apologise, I'll apologise even when I've done nothing wrong, it's like a form of tourette's syndrome.. Actually on that point, my language is fucking awful, I spend a lot of my time swearing, because I've got a Scottish accent it does actually fit the pattern of our speech really well. In fact opening a greeting to a mate as 'Alright ya fuckin' cunt' is actually quite an affectionate greeting, I love swearing, I feel a sense of freedom and being an independent adult when I swear, my friends will tell you I get in all sorts of trouble when I'm out in Glasgow, I have an example of this that I'd like to share. When I worked in Glasgow I'd find any excuse to go out, I have a great friend base and going for a cheeky wee after work pint was always an option. Anyways, one night we were out in a pub called 'Failte', I like it because it's like an old man's pub, run down, delapidated, stale etc, it's also a Celtic pub so you've got to watch what you say/discuss. So one night I was out with two of my closest friends (Heggie & Rab, absolute legends the pair of them, well.. Heggie is, Rab not so much, his patter can sometimes be pish..) and we were in Failte, now remember what I said earlier about the big voice? Couple that with three or four pints and it amplifies, well there were two old dears next to us, I'd hit the magical three/four pint mark and I started swearing like a fucking sailor, I was saying 'cunt' this, 'fuck' that and all the usual swears. (fucking is my favourite swear by the way) So very politely the two

old dears turned and commented that my language was a bit of an

abboration, now.. I'm a nice drunk, I've never been in a fight, I've never

been in trouble with the Police and I've never started any trouble, I'm also

have a lot of my wits about me, they normally deteriorate with the

increase in alcoholic consumption. So I politely apologised to the two

ladies, continued to drink and get drunk with my mates. A good 15-20

minutes slipped past, I had drunk more and I was basically back to being

loud and swearing. The two old dears said their goodbyes and headed for

the door, at the same time either Heggie or Rab done something, either

to my phone or my drink to which I shouted at them 'You pair of fucking

cunts!!' Of course, as my voice travels further than British Airways the two

old dears thought I'd shouted at them.. I...was...petrified, they came

storming back and before I had a chance to explain they were right there.

I was stammering and couldn't think, thankfully Heggie explained the

situation in a calm and rational manner (He is such a good drinker, you

NEVER know he's drunk, I envy him so much!) and then they left, I get

embarrassed really easily and my face went bright red, so needless to say

I took the brunt of abuse for the remainder of the night. I'm good that

way, I'm an entertaining drunk and my entertaining (but not known to myself actions) normally end up on Facebook. I fall asleep drunkenly and the next day I re-live /cringe at what had happened the night before. One of the best nights I ever had happened in 2007, I fell out with my good friend Pamela 'Ella' Geelan, you don't need to know the story, it was all my fault, I was a dick. Anyways, we went to a pub called Campus East, (it no longer exists, sniffle.. loved Campus East!) we got absolutely wrecked, I mean fucking absolutely steaming, my last train was at 23:48 and I left Campus East at about 01:30/02:00? Anyways, the only option I had was to get a taxi but I had another idea. (I get GREAT ideas when I'm drunk, we should talk...) I worked in the middle of Glasgow so it was like a five minute walk from the pub, I decided rather than fork out £50 for a taxi back to Falkirk I'd go back into work, get under my desk and have a few hours sleep, I mean, who would know right? This was a fucking masterplan, I'd save £50 and also get a good five hours sleep, what could possibly go wrong? Well, here's what went wrong. I staggered back to work, the first problem was that the doors to get in were all locked, there was a two foot gap I briefly attempted to get under and gave up, was quite skinny but not... that skinny. So there's a door and when the main gates are closed you can access via this door, I thought no problem, ah... but there was, there was also a security gate in front of the door and between that and the door was a gap of about one foot. The gate was about seven feet tall? I'm just about six foot so I couldn't jump it, I was drunk for fuck sake. There was a wee wall I could climb up so I figured if I could climb the wall and then jump inbetween the gate and the door I could then let myself in, great plan, what could possibly go wrong, I mean.. it's fucking foolproof right? Was it fuck. I jumped from the wall, misjudged the jump and ended up wedged between the security gate and the door, I was stuck, I was drunk and at first I thought it was well funny. After being stuck for TWO FUCKING HOURS I found it less funny, it was Winter, it was 04:00 and I was working in five hours, eventually some nice French students walked by and seen my predicament, the first question they asked was 'Are you ok?' Am I ok? Does it fucking look like I'm ok, I'm stuck in a one foot gap at 4am in the fucking morning, does this look like a man that's ok? Anyways that was internal monologue, I explained I wasn't and they rang for assistance, the security guard thankfully didn't recognise me and when he asked how it happened I said 'some friends through me over', funny eh? I couldn't very well detail the greatness of my master-plan could I? I ended up paying about £60 for the taxi home, had two hours sleep and then got up for work again, ooft what a hangover. The first mistake I made was to tell my friends, within about an hour it was everywhere and to this day, that's how a lot of people know me, my friends still tell this tale, I find it hilarious although at the time I thought, what a fanny. This is less funny but I also went to a strip-club, spent £260 (it was fuckin' braw!) got a taxi home and fell asleep in my chips and cheese, I didn't notice when I got in so when I got up in the morning I thought my eyes were playing tricks, they weren't, my forehead was a kind of yellow-cheese colour. Fail. So you see my life isn't all doom and gloom, I have some phenomenally good nights out and some fantastically good times, I'm a great guy to be around and that shows with the amount of friends I have, I make friends easy, I just sometimes struggle to keep them sometimes as I can be a bit of a fanny, on the rare occasions I've fell out with friends I can't think of one time where it's been their fault. I'm flawed but funny. I think that would be the hardest thing, people would have a lot of stories about me if I am to commit suicide. Although they'd remember me fondly they would always hate me for giving in to suicide. I know this but I don't know how much to tell them just how much I'm struggling with this, do I tell them or do I just... do it and get it over and done with. I don't know, I really don't. I just... I just don't know what to do, suicide is irreversible, once I take the step and do it, I'd need to make sure that I killed myself, the worst thing would be waking up in hospital surrounded by friends and family, I'd never be trusted on my own again, it would break the trust and faith shown in me by friends and family, they'd never allow me out their sight and even worse they may even put me in psychiatric care. That's why if I'm going to commit suicide I need to make sure I succeed. I need to not only have accepted the finality of it but I would need to commit to saying goodbye to everyone, no matter how much it pained me I know my pain would soon be over, for the people I hold closest their pain would only be beginning. Me and death have always been on the same page, I've never really felt afraid of dying, even when I was younger (14/15 years old) it often came into my head, there is one certainty in life when you're born and that is that you're going to die, it's fact, there's no disputing it, running away from it, hiding from it. Death comes to us all, the question is how we will meet our maker, some live a long, prosperous life and die peacefully, some people get life yanked from them by cancer, some people die in accidents and some people like me think of ways to quit early. I don't want anyone thinking for one second I'm glorifying suicide, you know 'leaving a beautiful corpse' and having people reminisce about the crazy bastard I was. This is just a story of someone who is bang in the middle of wanting to beat it and not sure if he has got the strength to get through the other side, I said this earlier but

I need to be clear, I think suicide is a selfish act, I always have done and regrettably I've seen a few friends in their 20's take their own life, I've cursed them, attended their funeral, cried and then hated them for doing it. I know it's wrong, I know it's selfish, I know it's the old saying of 'winners never quit and quitters never win' but I just don't feel like a winner, I very rarely have. Everything gets thought about all the time, I've spent the last 81 days (17/08/2014 to 06/11/2014) evaluating whether if this is the timing is right for me to say goodbye, I must be doing something right as I'm still here fighting it, my concern is that if I can't fight it anymore then I'll need to say goodbye, I don't even know how I would do it, I mean.. would I phone everyone, put a general post on Facebook, text everyone, gather everyone around and tell them I have no fight left and that I'm checking out forever. I honestly don't know how I would go about it but the fact that I am thinking about it means that I have question marks about my immediate future. As far as the doc , my work and my family/friends are concerned I'm beginning to recover. I am to an extent but I've always found it easy to put on a face to the people I speak to most, the truth is it's now 06/11/2014 and if anything I feel worse than when I started, the fact that suicide is the dominant thought in my mind means something just isn't working. I don't even know if I'll see Christmas, I don't even know if I'll be here in a week.. Ungrateful eh? Maybe if I talk about it that much that I'll get bored and just... move on with my life. Yea', right.. I've never really been good at anything I've done, sure I play golf, the odd game of five-a-side football, badminton but I'm not really that good, at golf I did play off six in my younger days which wasn't bad but I was practising like six times a week. I'm not even that good with a girl, I can't hold down a relationship, I go cold on people quite quick and in the bedroom I'm at best, average. I'm not short on manhood which is nice but it's almost like my life gets to a certain point and I hit the internal big red button to 'destroy everything', it's happened a few times, just when things have been going well and then BANG! It all blows up and I end up back on my own again. I genuinely like being on my own, (my dating profile would tell you otherwise, according to that I'm like the best guy that ever was, I do however grow a tremendous beard, it's awesome until it turns ginger, what the fuck?!) I don't know it's because I can fart and scratch my balls until I'm content but I genuinely feel a certain level of serenity when I'm on my own. (well.... when my mind isn't racing and causing me to think of suicide..) It's becoming a struggle, a real struggle. I was out with two good friends last night (07/11/2014, exactly nine years after I started with 3) and I had a good night, I drank though, only had four pints but it was enough for me to open up to them, I cried as I looked them both in the eye and said that I genuinely don't know if I'm going to make it through the other side of this, I told them that every day is a fight and it's a fight that I manage to get through every day. I love my friends because they accept me for who I am and they appreciate me at my worst, they see I'm at my worst and they're fully supportive of me. I went out last night wearing sunglasses, mainly because I can hide behind them, they almost make me feel like I'm invisible and I can hide my emotions from people. It didn't work last night, I cried a lot and said to my friends that I'm not just battling depression, I'm fighting off thoughts of suicide and that was a really hard thing to say, I actually said this may be the last time that I see them, this could be the last time I'm out, this could be the last time that I see my friends. I am doing everything in my power to get through this, I'm doing something that I've never done before and that's opening myself right up, I've been guilty in the past of just saying 'I'm ok' and that I'm having 'good days and bad days', I'm not having good and bad days, I'm having bad days, a LOT of bad days. I can count on two hands how many good days I've had since 01/09/2014, there's not a lot so when they come along I grab them and make the most of them. I have to, if I'm going to make it through this then I need to use every resource available. I need my friends, my family, my GP, employee support lines, I need everything, people need to know how hard I'm actually fighting this, they need to know that if I don't make it out the other side then at least I gave it 100%, at this point in time if I was to put a number on myself getting through it I'd say I've got a 40% chance of making it through. I want to get that number up and I want to live my life, I just want to live, that's all I want, I don't have big dreams or plans, I just want to get through my life, enjoy it and when it's time for me to go I can go. I feel so ungrateful for feeling like this, for wanting to end my own life early, it kills me every day and it's something I want to shake. I met a really good friend on Wednesday, we went to the cinema (I think the last time I was at the cinema was 2009? It was aaagggesss ago) and we watched a film, she said something that's very true and it was: "The past is a stick that we beat ourselves with" It's true, I mean it's absolutely bang on. What's the point on focusing on things that have happened in the past, you can't change them and you'll never be able to change them. It's all about being in the present and dealing with things as they come. I've done some awful things in the past, some things that I just cannot shake from my mind, they get replayed, analysed, re-played and then analysed again, I can't stop that from happening and I know that doesn't help me. It can't be healthy looking at things that have happened and beating yourself up over them. So if that's the case then why am I having so much trouble with leaving them where they belong, in the past and just... getting on with my life, what good is it doing me for me to keep re-playing events in my head? Back in 2006 I used to be a pretty good golfer, I played off six so I knew my way around a golf course, I played pretty well consistently because I was able to control my mind. (most of the time) I hit a pretty long ball off of the tee, my iron play was solid and the best part of my game was chipping and putting, that helped immensely because it knocked three to four shots off of my score every single time. When I was down to this level I had a trick for dealing with bad shots, I can't remember if someone told me or I read it in a magazine but the tip was if you hit a bad shot you take six steps, think about it and then you forget it. So what you're basically doing is not allowing one mistake to fuck up the rest of your round, you move to the next shot and then you concentrate on that, if you dwell on the bad shot you can then just... blow up and just ruin your round. I've been fortunate enough in my golfing life to break 70, (for an amateur this is an achievement) I played the round of my life, I was out in four under par and returned home four over par, I went round in 67 and I still have the scorecard from that day, I look back and every time I see it I smile. What that shows me is if I put enough effort into something and have control of my mind I can do anything I want to do. The lesson is I need to control my mind and not let my mind control me, that's what's happening just now, I'm... I'm.... I'm doing all of the right things but I just can't seem to turn the corner. Am I putting too much pressure on myself? Am I doing enough to help myself? Over this last week I have become really lazy, I am sleeping so much just now and my legs are actually hurting because I'm just... not moving. That's one of the worst things you can do because you think and over-think, in fairness that's what I do normally anyway, even when I'm feeling ok. I wish this was fuck off because it's fucking me right off...

I don't think there's any way for me to say this without sounding weird so I'll just come right out with. I humanise inanimate objects, I develop feelings for them and when I leave the house/walk past them I feel a tinge of sadness. That's weird eh? For example, before me and Steve moved to the house we're in just now (it's a very very nice house, two xBox One's, a pool table, PS4, it's spacious, warm and it's top floor overlooking a canal, it's a pretty awesome house. I also have a Sega Mega Drive which I still play way too much!) we stayed in quite a small flat, I mean it was tiny,

how we didn't fall out I didn't know, in fairness the only time that me and

Steve have fell out is when we carried a pool table up six flights of stairs,

that was a fucking awful day. In the old house we had a boiler in a

cupboard and it was a 'Potterton', I don't know if it's a good make or not

but I formed an attachment with Potterton, most times I walked past him

to heat the water for a shower I would touch the top of him in a sort of

comforting way, when I was leaving for work I would even open the door

and just... smile at him before I left for work, I mean, that even sounds

crazy just writing that but I humanise things, I form bonds with things that

have no feelings, sometimes before I leave this house I'll open the living-

room door and smile at the living room, knowing it's on it's own until I

come home. I'm sure that's not normal but it's true, sometimes I actually

feel bad for leaving the house because I think 'it'll be dark when I see you

again'. I mean I don't think I'm violating any laws or doing anything wrong

but should a man form relationships with inanimate objects? Is that what

a normal person does? Do any of you do that? I still miss 'Potterton', we

moved out on 27/06/2013 and I actually found it really hard to say

goodbye to him. I still think about him and I miss him, he was like.. a

support, something familiar that I knew, someone that I knew that could get me through a bad time if I was having one. Sitting here writing this I'm beginning to feel like I'm sounding a bit loopy, what's the point in writing something like this if you're not going to be honest, I need to be 100% honest otherwise writing this is a huge waste of time and effort. This all needs to come out so people can see exactly what goes on in my head and how much I've got to fight every day just to stay alive. People need to see that I'm not the person I proclaim to be and that I harbour a LOT of secrets, dark secrets that I'm almost too scared to write down because I fear I'll be carted off to the nearest mental hospital. I'm too scared to be myself, I'm too self-conscious of what other people think of me, I don't know why because 99% of people I come across aren't going to be in my life, so why am I so socially conscious? To give you an insight I've always been a colourful person, I like bright colours, I like tops that stand out and I don't like looking... normal. I've had blue mohawks, red mohawks, blue hair, red hair, green hair, that's probably why I've not got any hair now. (aww) I've had two lip piercings, my eyebrow pierced and I was twelve feet away from getting the old 'Prince Albert', thank fuck I didn't, that would have fucking hurt. Until the age of 30 I wore really baggy trousers and had more colourful tops than what the high street did, I had enormous headphones and I would blast Metallica, Bad Religion, Rise

Against from and generally I didn't give a fuck, well.. that was the picture I painted anyways. Deep down I was always really conscious of society's/friends opinions of me, I still am. Last night I went out with Heggie & Stuart McIwain (two of my best buds) and I wore a multi-coloured top, (it was like a packet of fruit pastilles) nice jeans, white trainers, yellow sunglasses and a tie, that was how I used to be and it felt so good to just stand out from everyone else, I wasn't conscious and I just.. had a good time as I was more myself, as the night went on and the alcohol flowed it did go downhill a bit, the reason for that though was that I had to tell my friends about my true feelings as mentioned previously, I feel better for doing it though, I'm not hiding behind it anymore, I'm actually staring it straight in the face and trying to make it blink before I do. That's all good stuff and I'm genuinely proud of myself for going out, I cancel plans like you wouldn't believe, I'm a selfish bastard and I only do things on my terms. That's not being a good friend but luckily I've got good friends who still see the good in me, even when I hit the self-destruct button and try to fuck things up. In our current house I haven't formed any real relationship with an inanimate object yet, weird considering we've been here for one year, four months and twelve days, I thought by now I'd be caressing the toaster or hugging the fridge but I'm not. I'm living a relatively normal life and not committing myself to a lifetime of inanimate bliss. I somehow felt with Potterton that he understood me, like he got who I was and he would actually make me feel better when I had my not so good days. While I'm writing this I still think of him in his wee cupboard keeping the water nice and warm and the flat nice and warm, he was a wee chunky so and so, if I had to define his shape I'd say he was curvy, I used to strategically lay the towels on top of him evenly so that he wouldn't be weighed down too much. When Steve left for work and I was on my own I would go out of my way to see Potterton, I'd spend a lot of time with him and I would talk to him when I had problems, so I did tell someone all of my problems but regrettably he couldn't give me any advice, he just hummed away, had his wee LCD display that showed you what temperature the water was at and his wee dials that you could alter the temperature with. If I can be honest with you I felt more comfortable around Potterton than what I did with friends, I know this is beginning to sound a little surreal and I want to assure you nothing happened between me and Potterton, we were just friends.. we were really good friends and I miss him. (sad face) When I talk to people about my problems I feel as if they're judging me or they think I'm making stuff up, I feel like they're not looking at me but they're looking straight through me, I don't know if that's true but it's just how I feel. When I worked in my old job I had more than one discussion with my manager about my mental state, she was so understanding and such a good boss, she completely got what I was saying and on my not so good days when I'd burst into tears she helped me. I appreciate all the help that she gave me and I repaid that by drinking a can of Jack Daniels & Coke at my desk before a night out, great eh? I openly sat there and drank alcohol, fortunately enough I got dragged over the coals and received a final written warning for my behaviour. My boss done the right thing and acted professionally, I then went to our night out and made an absolute tit of myself, I stood at the bar and didn't talk to anyone, what an arsehole, it was 29/11/2013 and I can safely say it was the worst working day of my life. I didn't handle myself at all well that day and to all that had to deal with me I'm super sorry, I didn't mean to be a dick but unfortunately it comes to me quite easily. I got a work referral to go and see a specialist, we discussed my past and why I thought I had done this and I simply stated 'I don't know', I didn't really want to open up to him, in hindsight I wish that I did because that was a real chance to get myself back on track. (Damn) I wish I could live a lot of my life retrospectively, I would change so much. In the moment I don't think clearly and when I look back at the event in question I always find a way that I could have handled it better. I find myself daydreaming a lot, I always have done and I don't know why. Even when I was 14, 15 and playing golf with my Dad I'd find myself looking up at the sky at a passing jet and walking past my golf ball. I would be miles away just wondering where the jet was off to, who was on it, what's their life story. Who's the pilot? Is this their last flight? Is it a woman? Is it someone going away to start a new life? From a young age I was quite inquisitive but it was internally, not externally which I think made a difference. If I'd been more open as a kid I think I could have turned out differently, I don't know if I would have but I don't think I could be any worse than what I am. A borderline alcoholic who's paranoid, insecure, balding and in real danger of throwing away his life. I've never really seen myself in a position of authority like a manager or anything, I just think I'd find a way to screw it up, I've always been a conscientious worker, on my high school report cards that was a recurring phrase, my teachers knew that I wasn't that smart but I would always apply myself, in my working life I'd say that is a fair assessment of me. I'm a team-player, I always have been. Whatever job I've done I've always thought of not only my actions but how my actions would affect my team. I'm all for digging in and getting stuff done, I work late when needed, change my shift when needed, get calls when there are queues and do anything my manager asks. I'm good at what I do, I have a good way with people, I know customer service inside out and I'm an asset to any employer, just sometimes I'm 'a little fiery' or I lose my temper and my headset gets flung halfway across the call centre, that's something I need to work on because it's not nice to see. I'm quite an angry person as well so I need to control that. In the rare times that I've looked at living past the age of 35 I've seen myself staying on my own in some modest flat in Larbert, still working in a call-centre and drinking heavily, I can see myself drinking a lot and putting on lots of weight, I can see myself distancing myself from my family and just.. dying alone, just severing ties with the world and slowly easing myself out of people's lives. That's sad eh? For a man to think like that is just... bad. Don't get me wrong I don't like it but I have an extremely low opinion of myself, that's one of the things I think that's holding me back from being a success, the fact that I don't have that killer instinct, that will to win and be better than everyone, I'm quite happy being mediocre, a face in the crowd, a worker. The less responsibility I have the less chance I have of making a cunt of things because I invariably would. I spend a lot of time trying to be in other people's minds, maybe I should have given psychology a go when I was younger. It blows my mind but there's approximately six billion people in the world and they all think individual thoughts, what do they think about daily, what do you think about daily? What goes through your head, what do you want to ultimately achieve in life, I'm fascinated, I'm in, I want to learn more about people and what makes them tick. That's something I'm happy to admit to, people interest me, I can sit in a pub on my own and just people watch, for hours, well until I get drunk and then I see two of everyone, (Aw) I look for any signs of emotion or any micro-expressions like fear, anger, joy etc. It's the same when I'm commuting, although it looks like I've just got my earphones in and reading the paper I'm actually studying everyone that comes on to the train, where they sit, how are they looking today and are they ok. I say this word a lot in my professional life but I do genuinely 'empathise' with people, I feel a lot and I'm not talking about goosing people or anything, I feel so much in my body, when someone is crying on the train or they look as if they're having a hard time I just want to hug them. There was one time I was commuting to Edinburgh, it was the middle of summer, the train was hot and over-crowded, I was feeling really low and surprisingly I was weighing up the pros and cons of suicide, I had some low mood music on and I was daydreaming out the window when suddenly this guy just.. collapsed, he took a really sore one and banged his head on the door, he collapsed with what looked to be heat exhaustion, after a few of us attended to him and made sure he was ok we then alerted the train staff, I don't know how the rest of his day was but I know mines definitely picked up, I was ok and this poor guy had collapsed. I was having some lunch later in the day, think it was a Pot Noodle, (I have a thing for chicken and mushroom Pot Noodles, yum..) all I could think about was this guy on the train, how long had he been feeling unwell, was there an underlying condition or was it just the hot, cramped train that caused him to just.. collapse. I genuinely hope he's ok because he took a really nasty fall, amazing how one event can just... change your mindset for the rest of the day. I wish I could talk to people, like if I was a counsellor or a psychologist, that'd be a dream job for me because of my intrigue for the human mind. I'd love to get to the root of people's problems and feel like I've made a difference, I'm pretty sure I'm seeing a psychologist in a few weeks and I've got hundreds of questions for him. He looks like a pretty cool guy, I hate to admit this but I judge a lot on looks when it comes to my mental state, if I don't like the look of someone I won't give them anything except the basics, luckily I've always had good professionals looking after me and my local GP is amazing, I'm so thankful to him for all that he's done for me. I'll need to find a way to thank him for all his efforts, he's been immense and provided so much help. If I do get through this I want to try and help fellow sufferers of depression and try to turn people's lives around, I don't think anyone should fight alone, I've accepted I can't beat this on my own and I'm taking all the help I can, this is the first time I've actually taken antidepressants, if you'd mentioned them to me previously I would say no, I was too caught up in the side effects and not the good they do. Unfortunately my current tablets aren't really doing anything for me, I don't feel more stable, I don't feel any change in mood, I just.. feel the same every day, I'll really need to speak to my GP about that. I do want to help people though, I'll start looking into this and talk it through with my family tomorrow, I want to do something to be remembered by in life, I don't want to just.. fade away with a dreary funeral and people being angry at me for committing suicide, I want a purpose to live, I want to do something worthwhile and if I can help at least one person I'll be happy, if I can impact someone else's life and change their outlook on depression I'll take it. Depression is such a horrible illness, I've always felt as if I'm not really ill when I've been of f work with it, because there's no physical illness I almost feel like I'm skiving, you can't underestimate the importance of your mental health though, it's such a critical part of life and should be treated with the same respect as looking after yourself physically. The more I'm writing this the more I'm fearing what's going to come out, I feel as if I'm procrastinating and if I don't say what's happening in my mind it's like it's not happening? I think there is a right time and place for what's going to be said and I think the next chapter is the best place for me to say it, I'm sorry if what it contains disturbs you, I apologise if what I say causes alarm but the reason for writing this was to get this out, it's to get out what I dare not say this to a professional, it's the part of my mind that no-one else has seen, you are going to be the first to witness this, you are going to be the first people that are going to know this about me. I think

So, I think it's safe to say that 'introductions' are over, you can see into my head and see what goes on in it, you see what makes me tick and now I feel comfortable enough to let you in, if you're ready to see what's really inside my head, read on. I warn you though, this is going to be absolutely brutal, this is going to be no-holds barred, shackles off. This is me completely exposing myself to you, so if you're ready, let's begin.

Well, here it comes, here's everything that I've been fearing, everything I've been hiding and running away from. All that's gone before feels like I've been sparring, now I'm fighting for real. So, as you now know I've suffered a lot with depression, what no-one knows is just exactly what I think daily, it's horrifying, truly horrifying. Here goes... I have a great family and friends, I've mentioned it one hundred times before and they know I love them. The hardest part of what goes on in my mind is I regularly think about killing people, family, friends and pets. I think the level of trust I have is one I can easily abuse. I don't know why I think like this, I don't know why I think these thoughts because all they do is upset me and cause me to cry. It's almost like they've been burned in to the front of my mind, I don't know how it started, I don't know why it happens but what I do know is I think about killing... A LOT. I think of ways that I could totally just kill people and then kill myself like a coward, I think of ways that I can kill people like using a baseball bat, suffocating them, beating them to death or torturing them. This I know for certain is not normal, all my life I've felt I was different but this I know is insanity, it's ridiculous and the scary thing about it is I think these thoughts most days, I don't have any intention of killing anyone but for some reason, I look at knives, ovens, pans, golf clubs, I look at anything I could use as a weapon and think about how I could inflict pain on the people I love the most. That terrifies me so much because I'm one of the nicest people you'll ever meet, I'm social, affable and generally just.. a good guy, to actually read this back it just.. makes it real what I think, I don't know if this makes me a psychopath, if it means I'm just troubled or if I'm just fucked up. It causes me not to sleep at night, it causes me to neglect my personal hygeine as I'm worried that I'm gearing up for murder, it's almost like if I don't take care of myself I'm working against my thoughts. I feel physically sick at what I'm writing because once it's out there, it's OUT THERE. I don't know how people would react . I can't stop anyone from reading this, I can't stop people from thinking what they think of me but one thing I'll be glad of is that people can see the person that I actually am. I don't want any applause for what I'm saying but the fact I fight these thoughts off regularly I feel is testament to the sheer amount of mental strength that I have, for me to think these thoughts, process them, analyse them and then conquer them shows a tremendous amount of self-control. I've learned to deal with them in the same way as my depression, I have things that I do when they start, for example I'll run a hot bath, turn all the lights out, put some music on and just... lay in the bath until they.. disappear. When I play golf I imagine that the ball represents all of my negative thoughts and it focuses me on swinging through and knocking it miles. I play my xBox and when I'm playing an RPG (Role Playing Game) I imagine all the bad guys being bad thoughts and each kill is a bad thought defeated. Gaming is a tremendous form of escapism, ironically killing people digitally stops me from the thought of me killing people in real life. Now as you're reading this I have no idea what you think of me, I don't want to influence that, I want to lay bare everything that's in my head and at the end you can make your own decision on what I am. I want to completely expose myself and my mind and I want people to dissect it, discuss it, debate it. I want people's opinions, I want feedback whether it be positive or negative, I want to meet people and openly discuss my problems and their problems, I want everything to be out in the open so there are no hiding places, writing this gets every single thing in my head out and on to paper, something that's terrified me for the last seven to eight years. I've always felt if this was kept inside then I'd find a way to defeat it. I always thought that no-one needed to know this, given the way that things have been over the last eight weeks it's become blatantly obvious that this needs to be out, not just for me to see but for everyone to see. I want to open my mind and let the guts of it just pour out, I do have reservations about it though because this is the first time that I've shared this with anyone, my GP doesn't know

and my family and friends definitely don't know this. I'm not sure I'd ever

be able to tell my family about this, the same way I will never say to them

I'm thinking of committing suicide, I don't think I could do it, I can see

their faces, it would break them to know I was thinking it, it would break

them if I done it. I'm not trying to pass myself off as some poor boy that

needs a cuddle or sympathy, I need to dig and dig until it all comes out

and this weight lifts off of my shoulders. The demons I encounter are

pretty wild, they're vicious, they're evil and they weigh me down as if I'm

wearing armour weighted with the demons, somedays I can't even look

straight ahead, I can only look down as if they're forcing me to. I was

actually doing ok until Robin Williams died, he committed suicide and he

had struggled with it, I started thinking will I ever beat this, I started

thinking if he was in his sixties and he done it, could I posslbly live my

whole life and not give in to suicide? That started it, that started me

thinking and when I start thinking all that happens is more thoughts pile

on, my mind gets faster, I can't cope, I start drinking a lot and then I

collapse. I hate myself, I absolutely fucking hate myself, it would be better

if I just done it, people would have one less person to worry about and

the world would wash it's hands of a loser. A true fucking loser, the world doesn't need people like me, people that are the black sheep of society, dragging them back so that they can hold my hand and tell me I'm going to be ok, I'm not deserving of anyone's support, I wish they'd cut me away, I wish I would have the balls to do something about it, I want to run away, start a new life, forget everything there is to know about Dave Roberts and just die cold and alone, secretly that's what I want, it must be. You can't right this kind of stuff if you're happy in your own mind, please friends and family cut me loose, I'll not drag you down any more, I won't hold you back, I won't take up your time with my selfish needs, maybe if I do something horrible then people can just forget me, maybe people can see what is inside me and burn it away, kill it with fire. I need to cleanse this, I need to beat this, I need to fucking beat this, I WANT TO FUCKING BEAT THIS, I'VE HAD ENOUGH, I CAN'T FEEL THIS WAY ANY MORE, I NEED HELP, I AM REACHING OUT FOR HELP, I AM STANDING UP AND SHOUTING 'I.. NEED HEEEEELLLP, HEEEEELLLPPPP ME PLEASE, FOR THE LOVE OF GOD SOMEONE GIVE ME SOMETHING TO STOP THIS PAIN, DRUG ME, PLY ME WITH BOOZE, TORTURE ME, BEAT ME, DO WHATEVER YOU NEED TO SO I CAN START LIVING AGAIN, HELP ME AND I'LL HELP YOU, I MEAN IT, I'LL HELP YOU ANYWAY I CAN... My heart rate is through the roof, my eyes are wide open, I'm breathing so quickly and so shallow, that's all come out, that felt good, oh.. that... felt.. GOOD. My heart honestly feels like it's coming out my chest, my breathing is becoming slower, my heart rate is slowing down, was that it? Was that what I needed to come out? Was this the thing that was causing my suffering. I feel like I've just had the best orgasm of my life, all I need is a cigarette and I'd be happy, I feel, like a massive weight has just been taken off my shoulders, I feel lighter, I feel cleaner, I feel better for shouting at the top of my voice what I said up there, I still read it and it causes my pupils to dilate, it looks good, oh.. it feels sooo fucking good. After four rounds of sparring I've got down to business and I've came out swinging. I am so proud of myself for putting all of that down, I'm so proud of myself for saying it, for writing it. I want to call my friends and family and tell them I no longer want to hurt them. Oh, wait, I can't do that because I haven't told them this. Oh.. errmm... well I'm still proud of doing it, whether it confines me to a mental institution or not at least I know I've managed to dig deep enough to get it out, you've no idea how good a feeling it is to say that, it's like a shackle has been broken, where did that come from? Was that why I started writing this, this chapter, was this what I wanted to let the world to know? Was this what was holding me back, bringing me down, was this the thought cluster that caused all of the other problems?

I'll be honest I don't know. What I do know is that it's 08/11/2014 and it's 20:54, I'll never forget this time and date, this was the first time I reached way down in myself and I pulled the demons out by their throat and slayed them right on this page, I managed to do that on my own and with no alcoholic influence, as a reward I'm going to treat myself to a cup of tea. Everyone has their own demons that they face, some people go through life relatively unscathed, some people are successful, some people face demons and beat them and unfortunately some people succumb, personally I don't think my demons will ever completely disappear, they are always going to be there for the rest of my life, regardless if I beat this or not, the point I was keen to make to my friends last night was I am throwing the kitchen sink at this, I'm giving it my all in the hope that I see that corner and I can turn it, after what I've written above I feel like I've smashed through a barrier, a barrier that's been getting bigger and bigger for the last seven to eight years, I feel like I've achieved something, I feel emotions that I've not felt for a long time, I feel a sense of relaxation, I feel contented, I feel a sense of fulfilment in what I've managed to draw out of my mind for you to see. My head is actually sore from what's come out, it actually feels like the demons have been pulled out the front of my head , it feels like every part of my body is lighter, as if this came from my toes, it's a feeling I never want to dissipate, it's a feeling I want to keep forever, I know I can't so I'm going to enjoy it while I can. For the first time in years I'm actually looking forward to going to my bed tonight, I feel like I could sleep for weeks, I apologise if you feel I'm over-emphasising this but this for me is the breakthrough I've been looking for, this is the culmination of all that time where I've wanted to be alone, where I've suffered, the time where I nearly committed suicide in 2011. I feel like I've learned from that and for the first time I think that I might beat this! I really hope that I do and I hope that this feeling I have stays with me. Now I've got through that I can now talk to you about my near suicide in 2011, I didn't handle it at all well, I was feeling good or so I thought. I'd started seeing a girl but one of my friends and me fell out about it, she was much younger than me and I just.... flipped for some reason, in the space of three days I went from top of the world to posting a picture of me saying goodbye on Facebook, tears streaming down my face, I had six cans of Stella and a kitchen knife, I'd decided when the sun went down, I was going to slit my wrists and that would be it. Can I explain what flicked that switch, what caused me to just lose all lust for life and kill myself? No, I can't, I remember going out after work, I drink alone, I drink alone a lot, I don't think that's healthy. I got steaming drunk and argued with my mate about this girl, drunken text

arguing is lethal, there were things said that just.. shouldn't have been

said. Anyways, this happened on the Tuesday and two days later I went

out drinking in Glasgow again, I got really drunk, had a good night but the

amount of alcohol I'd consumed wasn't normal, I was pished, I was facing

the Friday with a third straight hangover. I done it and then stupidly I

agreed to not only go out drinking but with the person I'd fell out with,

why did I do this? Did I want to shortcircuit my mind and go loopy? Was I

fucking insane? I remember having three pints and then leaving, I left the

pub crying my eyes out and looking around Glasgow for the last time, this

was it. I was committing suicide and that was all there was to it. I cried on

the train, I cried buying the beer, I only stopped crying when I was alone

on my bed, my phone never stopped ringing, I had texts flying in from

everyone and I ignored them. I had the knife, I had the beer, as far as I

was concerned I had said my goodbyes and that was the end of it, I had

accepted suicide, I'd made peace with it, I mean.... that's fucked up right?

I'd made the choice to end my own life and to this day I don't know what

caused it. Luckily for me I had my Uncle as a friend on Facebook and he'd

called my Dad, the two of them almost knocked down the door they were

hitting it that hard, I answered, went to my bedroom and just... sobbed, I sobbed uncontrollably and I'll never forget the look on my Dad's face, I still see it, I see him standing next to the door and he was just.. horrified at what he was saying, my Uncle took the knife away and they took away the beer. There was then an update to everyone that I as ok and I hadn't done it, my phone didn't stop ringing, at one point I ran out of memory on my phone. I remember sitting in my living room with my Dad and Uncle when my Mum came running in, I lost it, I mean, I just.. crumbled instantly, I've always been close to my Mum, I love her so much and just the sight of her, her seeing me like THAT, I couldn't take it. I cried for ages, my stomach hurt because I cried that much. I explained to her about an incident with her Ford Escort car that happened in 2005, there was major damage to it, the reason for that? I had six pints of beer and then decided to drive. I fell asleep, careered into a lamp post and woke up just as I was veering onto the pavement, it's worth pointing out there were houses not even fifty feet from the edge of the road, I.. fell.. asleep whilst driving drunk, I should have died.. I got the car back home in the morning, I stayed at my girlfriends house that night, as I was drunk and couldn't see the damage I fell asleep. I went out the next morning and the car... was.. fucked. I parked it up at my Mum's house, went in as if everything was normal and didn't say a word, I waited for her to see the car and then I went out and gasped in horror, I denied knowing anything about it, I lied to my Mum, I carried that about for six years, I told her right there and then, when she was cuddling me on my sofa what I'd done, I apologised, I apologised a lot, my Mum forgave me, I don't know why, to this day I still look back and I wish that I'd died that night. After my parents left my brother stayed with me, I slept, I slept a lot, for the next week I just slept on my couch, I was exhausted, I was drained, it took me a month to even look at going back to work, it was almost like my entire conscience was cleared and I had a clean slate to start from. Did I mention I had good family? I have great family, I'll always be indebted to them, not just for that night but what they've done for me all of my life, they're my heartbeat, my oxygen, my blood, they're the reason I fight this, I want to spend as much time around them while they're here, god knows I'll miss them when they're gone. For the first time ever in my fight against depression I was able to tell my Mum & Dad what was going on, it was three weeks ago and I talked to them, I told my Mum I didn't want them worrying about me, I was fighting it and that was all they needed to know. My Mum hit the nail right on the head when it comes to who I am, I remember exactly what she said, it was: "You always portray yourself as a confident person but you're not" I couldn't have put it any better Mum, that is 100% who I am, I act like I'm this superconfident man when really I'm a shy, insecure boy. I need to start being the person I am and not the person I want to be, there's only so much you can put on a face before it comes apart, I want everyone to see me for who I am. I need them to see me for who I am. This year has been a year of firsts, as well as talking to my parents and being 100% honest with my GP I held nothing back when I went in to meet my boss at work. I had a meeting with HR and my manager, I laid everything bare, I sat and poured everything that I could out, I talked openly about my mental state, my past, current thoughts and current problems, I even said to them that 'I'm not sure I'm going to beat this, I'm trying but I can't guarantee I'll come out the other side'. I don't know if I should have said that to be honest but me going and being all coy and protective isn't going to help me, if ever there was a time for me to be totally honest, it's now. If I can't be honest in the greatest fight of my life when will I be? I only get one shot at beating this, this is the only time that I've felt prolonged depression, we're in November and I don't even know when I'm going to be able to go back to work, every time I make it from Wednesday to Wednesday to see my GP I feel I've achieved something, I've had seven days and I've made it through to see him again. I've went the whole week and whatever demons I've had I've managed to stave them off for another short while. The fight is never-ending, my mental strength is depleted at times but every day I can get through means it's another day I've survived, it's another day where I've looked to the future, I've looked to my friends and family and I've told them that I'm fighting, I'm fighting with all my heart and my head, it shows them I still care about them more than I care about myself and that's a good thing. Throughout this whole journey I've never stopped thinking of others, I have to, I'm an important part of people's lives, that's not meant to come out as arrogant as it does, I play a huge part in my friends lives and they would hate me if I gave in. They'd be fucking right too, what a selfish prick Dave was, just.. gave in.. He gave in, he tapped out, he quite, what a loser. I don't want people thinking that of me, I want to do things on my terms, so if I can get through to the end of the year and to my birthday (January 15) I'll view that as a massive achievement, I'll look at that and pat myself on the back. Do you see what I'm saying? Do you feel what I'm feeling? In no way, shape or form am I looking to commit suicide, I'm looking at doing every single thing I can to beat it. I've got myself through it before, I've kicked down the door of depression many times in the past and I'm looking to kick through this one. This time it's different because the mental strength has been waning, what is my strongest asset has been my biggest liability this time. I'm 100% confident that if I get back in control of my mind I can fight this and beat this, I can go out with my friends again, I can get drunk and post ridiculous posts on Facebook, I can make wonderful new friends like Thomas J Moore and Fiona Anne Moore, Rose Dallas, Pete Lindsell, Lisa Robertson, Andy Crawford, Jason McColm, Polly Elliot-Pyle and Fay Richie. I want to go back to having parties at my house, getting the pool table out, getting the mega drive out and just having a good time again. I want to play golf in the summer with my Dad, I'm at my happiest when I'm with him, (for a 67 year old he still hits a good ball!) I want to walk our wee puppy Misha, I want to see her grow and become the new family friend, I want to get on with my work, I want to expand myself and meet new people, whether it be on the back of writing this book I don't care, I want to have more confidence in myself, I should have more confidence in myself, I've got a lot going for me, I want to be a better person, I want the world to actually see me, I want the world to accept me for the nutjob that I am. I want to spend the rest of my life making friends and then when it's time for me to go I can go in complete peace. That's what I want, that's my dream, I want to be better around people, I want to understand people, I want to achieve, I want to dream again, I wish I was the person I was at 16, I was full of hope, if you'd said to me at 16 here's what you're like at 32 I would ask what the fuck went wrong, what happened? Did someone die? Did I marry and my wife died? What happened between 16 & 32 that caused me to go so far off course? If I could go back I'd approach many situations differently, I wouldn't have cheated on the girlfriends that I had, I'd like to apologise to them, I was an arsehole, I'm still a bit of an arsehole but if I could have a second chance I'd worship the very ground they walk on. I should have a girlfriend, I'm good enough, I just get to a point and then... blow up, I ruin it or I cheat. If I can get through this I can meet a nice girl, wine her, dine her and then settle down, I want to settle down, I want to be at peace with myself instead of constantly fighting everything. Writing this is actually really good therapy, why did I not do this before, why didn't I sit down and just write, why didn't I just write everything down that was troubling me, was I scared? I used to write songs/poems, in total I think I've written 500+ but in 2011 I threw them all out, I didn't want to look back at them. I'm glad I did but I still have one book, it was written in 2007 - 2009 and contains a picture of me and my family on the inner cover, it's an important book to me and it goes everywhere with me. I look back to that because it shows what I went through and it showed hope, it still gives me hope that I can beat this, although I don't want to beat myself up about the past I don't want to forget it either, I can see a lot of the demons circling in that book, it's cover-to-cover with painful writings but there are a few pages of hope in there somewhere. (and rants) The fact there's a picture of my family on the inside cover is huge, that was put there deliberately by me so I can look at it when I needed strength, I look at my Mum, my Dad and my brother and I smile, everyone is so happy, including me. I think I like that the most, the fact that I'm actually smiling. I don't smile a lot unfortunately, maybe I should try? I mean, what harm can it actually do? It can't make me feel any worse than what I feel just now right? I am exhausted , this has been a particularly exerting chapter to write, I've had to dig so deep to pull this out and it's catching up with me. The time is now 22:12 on 08/11/2014, I've written as much as I can today, I need sleep, I crave a decent night's sleep so I can come out swinging tomorrow, I want to let you in more now, I want you to see who I am and I want you to know it all. I'm going to bed for the night though, I.. am.. absolutely... fucking.. shattered. Night.

It took me a while to fall asleep last night, I kept thinking about what I'd written and what I'm uncovering on this journey, the sleep I did get was deep but contented, I went to bed and for the first time in a long while I lay in comfort and I lay relaxed. My sleep was weird, I recall dreams, I see dreams that I've had from years ago and I still think about them. The dream I had last night made absolutely no sense, I'm still trying to figure it out. Here's how it went: I was working in an office, it wasn't a regular office, it was like my current place of work but the layout was different, it was a smaller office, everyone was all over the place and my vision was blurred, that wasn't the worst part. I was naked, I recognised my own body shape and it was me, buck naked walking through the office, it then changed up a gear. I then went from being in an office to working about 500 feet in the air, it was outside and I was the only person this high up, my chair was stationed on a platform barely big enough for a computer and it kept wobbling, I kept teetering over the edge, I didn't like it, I felt sick. I then fell, I started falling towards the ground, was this death? Was this the dream where I don't wake up before I reach the bottom? Yes, yes it was, I smacked the ground so hard, I felt it in my face, it hurt.. but I wasn't dead, I landed a few feet away from a colleague, I couldn't see his face, I couldn't see his shape, he called for an ambulance. I then 'woke up' in my dream, I was on a street, I had a huge beard, I had hair, I saw three paramedics, two men and a woman, I was bloody, I was disorientated and the sun burned my eyes, it was soooo bright. I hated it. I passed out again and the next thing I was back on the 500 foot platform, I fell again but this time I didn't hit the ground, it then moved to me being sedated by about seven people, apparently I was some kind of monster, they stuck a massive needle in my arm, I screamed and then passed out again. The last part of the dream was the most surreal though. I was myself again, I had clothes on, I was walking normally and one of the people that sedated me smiled at me as I just... walked out the door. The dream closed with someone else falling off of the 500 foot platform, I don't know how it ended for them, the dream stopped and I was just.. asleep. I don't know what that means, I'm not an expert in deciphering dreams but I do recall one I've had on more than one occasion. I'm blind-folded, I can hear a low clamour of voices, I go up stairs and I'm then instructed to jump off a ledge, it's three foot high and there's a guy who does this massive karate kick as I'm dropping off the ledge, he connects and I die, that's it, my lights go out, I'm dead. I've had this dream about four times and each time it's the same, nothing changes in it, there's no change in the steps, I don't see any of the characters, I don't even see my executioner, I jump from the ledge, looking straight ahead and the last thing I see is my killer doing a 360 degree jump, hitting me in the face and I die. Weird eh? That one last night was weird but thankfully I've only had it the once, also I've not had the recurring dream for a while, to have the same dream on four seperate occasions has to have some significance, it has to mean something, surely? I've never told anyone about this dream, I don't think it's something that I can get an answer to, I don't know if anyone could decrypt it. It's strange how I can remember dreams vividly, it's just something I've accepted, I sleep pretty deeply, I also have nightmares as Steve will testify to, (sorry Steve!) I must be awful to sleep next to, mind you it's been that long since I've slept next to someone I'm thinking of getting one of those blow-up dolls, it's been twenty-two months since I last had someone in my bed, it's been twenty-two months since I last had sex. On a plus side my right wrist is definitely stronger than it was... I'm way too hard on myself, I've always been the same, I set myself impossibly high standards and every mistake I make I view it as a failure, I beat myself up, I curse myself and I just... over-analyse. I think about every word that I speak, did that sentence sound right? Was my tone inflection correct? Did I emphasise the right words? Could I have said that with more conviction? EVERY, sentence, EVERY word that I speak gets analysed, I don't switch off, I can't switch off. I want to switch off. I need to switch off. Why can't I relax though? I mean why can't I do a shift at work, come home and just... relax? Why do I feel the need to drink to relax? Remember what I said about 'the six steps' earlier when I was talking about golf? There was a time where I could do that with balancing my work life and my personal life. In the morning as soon as I got to work and I got through the door my personal things were forgotten, vice versa as well when I finished work, work brain switched off and the personal brain switched on. I done it pretty well and it helped, it really did. I was able to balance my personal life and my work life, dare I say it I was happy because I was managing, somewhere along the line though I lost the ability, the two then merged and my brain was cooked again, it was burnt out because it was just constantly on. I hate it, I like myself but I hate my mind, I curse my mind because it distorts and pollutes my thoughts, it can take a happy thought and mangle it beyond all recognition. I genuinely believe I have two persona's that I've got to manage, the happy side of me takes no management, I'm happy, things flow, words flow, I flow and I'm happy and confident, there is no effort required and I can think clearly. Then there's the other side, it takes so much to control it, to keep it down, to interact with society when all I want to do is stand in the middle of the street and scream, I want to yell out loud and expel all the sadness and hurt that lives inside me, it needs so much brain power, I'm physically exhausted at the end of the day, I get headaches, I go to bed and I just.. lie

and think, I think, I over-think, I still keep thinking. (Dave, STOP thinking,

please stop thinking, hit the lightswitch, find the switch, hit it and go to

sleep, I'm tired, I'm so fucking tired.. please, I beg you, switch off) I get up

for work and I can't... I can't pick myself up, I'm exhausted and I've got to

do it all again, I've just went through a twelve round boxing match, I'm

cut, I'm bruised, I'm sore, I ache and then I've got another one right on

top of it, I've got to fight again, it's another twelve rounds, god it's

another twelve rounds, you've got to be joking, I've got to do another

twelve rounds? I can't see, I can taste blood, I can't lift my arms, I want to

go down, throw in the towel, please.. let me throw in the towel, I quit, I

can't fight any longer, it's too much, I've had enough, I don't recognise my

own face anymore, my senses are distorted, which way is the exit, where

am I in the ring, who the fuck am I even fighting? Knock me out, finish it,

kill the pain, I can go in peace, my lights can turn off for good and that's it,

I'll die, I'll die. I don't though, I keep fighting, I keep hanging in there, I pull

myself up, I regain my vision, I summon strength from deep inside and I

rise to my feet, I sit in my corner and everything starts coming back, my

desire, my fight, my life, I want to fight this, I'm going to beat this, I need

to beat this, I WANT.. TO BEAT THIS, I want to punch it in the face and never stop punching it in the face, I want to wreck it, I want to smash it, I

want to have twelve rounds of inflicting nothing but pain, I want to do

another twelve rounds, I want to do ANOTHER twelve rounds, I want to

do twelve by twelve fucking rounds, I want one-hundred and forty four

minutes of me punching it's fucking lights out. I want to keep fighting it

until it's laying bloody and dead in the middle of the ring, I can stand over

it, look at it and say 'I've beaten you, I... have BEATEN you, I'm better now,

I'm the champ, I'm the greatest since Ali, I'm the mother-fucking

champion. That's the dream, that's what I'm striving for, I'm working

towards the day where I can slay my demons, it's a daily fight, it's an

hourly fight, I've got to fight it on the bad days, I spend every minute

fighting it, I've got to stop looking over the balcony, I need to stop looking

at the pills, the knife, the train, I need to get through this, I need to reach

DEEP down inside myself and summon, I need to summon and summon

and summon until I find that strength, yank it out and beat them for

another day. Fifteen years I've been doing this, fifteen long, bloody years

of fighting, it's had me on the ropes once, it lined me up for the TKO, it

started swinging and thankfully I was pulled. My Dad & my Uncle stopped

the fight, I accepted the loss but I didn't give in, I fought as hard as I could

and three years later I'm in an even worse fight but I'm holding my own, at the moment I'd say I'm slightly behind on points but I want to make them up, it's the ninth round and I'm beginning to get a second wind, I need to use it, I need to start punching.. I want to start punching again. I need to stop being so harsh on myself, I do. I need to learn to relax and just switch off, it's not good for you to constantly be on the edge, on tilt, it's not good for your head and it's definitely not good for your mind, trust me.. it's really not good for your mind! I look to anything I can to inspiration and normally I find a piece of music that appeases me, I find music that appeals to me and gently soothes me, my bath in total darkness relaxes me, I feel the beat of the music getting bigger in my chest, my heartbeat gets replaced with the drumbeat, I begin to breathe in time with the music, I allow the music to consume me, envelope me, take me to where I need to go, it allows me to escape, I break free, the water's hot and comforting against my skin and the music is the same against my mind. I lie there, I just lie there, eyes closed, I don't move, I let everything just disappear, the music banishes it, the music overpowers it and dispells it, I do that for half an hour and when I finally come out I don't feel as bad as what I did, it may only be temporary but it works, it really does work. It won't be the last time in my life where a bath and music might just save it. I have a thing called a 'Star-Master', it's a cool wee thing where it projects bright colours and shapes onto the ceiling, as I close my eyes I see them, they go really really fast and then really really slow so it's important to pick the right music or it totally defeats the purpose. My bath can be so important in life, once I get to the point of no return it helps me to just... relax, you know, calm down a bit. (It's ok Dave, ssshh, relax, relax and breathe, One... two, one... two., One.........two, One.......... and..... two, ssshhh, it's ok, it's ok, listen to the music, listen to the words, guitars, listen to the drums though, the drumbeat, the heartbeat in the song, it's in your chest now, can you hear it beating? Keep it, keep it there and one... two, one...... two, one........ two and one......... and............. two, in... and... out, sshhhh, it's ok) Then and only then do I find that rare moment of peace, that moment of tranquility that I've been searching for the last day, two days, week, month. There it is, I've found it, all is well, my breathing slows, my bones relax, I allow my body to go limp and I just float around the house, I can look outside and not look over the balcony, I can see the trees, I see Stirling in the distance, I see a church, I see swans, birds, cars, people, bikes, joggers and runners. I feel normal again, I don't feel the pain, I feel appeased and at ease. Have I beaten it again? Have I conquered them again? It feels like I have, I'm going to go to sleep, I put some soft music on and I allow myself to drift, I don't think about the bad, I think about seeing my friends the next again day, should I buy them donuts? I feel generous, I'm feeling good so I'll do something good. Sure enough the next day I get up, I can look at myself in the mirror, I put my best foot forward and I attack the day, it's a great feeling the first day after the storm, everything is so calm and so nice, it's like the spring in my mind. The birds singing in the trees and the sun beaming down a gentle heat, the birds that left for the winter fly back home because they know there's good weather ahead. I like that, I really feel at ease the first day after the fight, I just... I love everyone, I could hug random strangers, I don't mind if Scotrail are late, (I'm fucking used to it anyway with them, run a train service? They couldn't even run a fucking bath, god I hate them..) I don't mind that my train is over-crowded, it's fine. I've got my music, I'm going to see the people I love and I'm going to go to work and help people with their various problems in a calm and professional manner. I don't mind customers, I get why they're angry, it's my job to look at things both from a customer's side and the business side of things, I'm pretty good at sorting things out for people, I'm friendly to them, I use their name and I try to speak to them the way I like to be spoken to. I phone customer service rarely and when I do I'm always super-polite because I realise they have a very hard job, dealing with the general public is, they expect service, they want things done yesterday and quite rightly, if there weren't customers with your respective business you wouldn't have a job, it's as simple as that. I like working in a call-centre, I set my various programs up the same way every morning, I like to have everything in order before I start, I'm meticulous, my desk layout never changes, my coffee sits in the same place on my desk every day, I have my headset volume at six bars, I always ensure I'm logged in bang on my start time, I'm never late, well the times that I am late are normally down to Scotrail/Scotfail, I REALLY, REALLY don't like using them, the thing that gets me about them is they are the only train firm in Scotland and when I'm off my cramped, late journey the conductor says 'Thanks for travelling with Scotrail today', as opposed to what? Taking a bike along the track? Flying Easyjet? Walking? Using one of those old-timey pump handle trains where the two of you work a lever and effectively push yourself to work? I'm going to walk away from this because if I stay on Scotrail I'll end up writing about one-hundred thousand words and I don't want to do that. I think you see what my feelings for them are so I'll leave them and hopefully I won't have to mention them again. I've been thinking about something I said earlier, it's been buzzing around my mind since I've written it: "You can't see where you're going if you're always looking back" It's true, have you ever dare tried to walk down a street whilst looking back? Not only would your neck be sore you'd never get to where you're going, in order for me to make my ten-minute walk from home to the train station I need to look forward, if I look back I'll crash into things or be killed, I need to cross a main road, that just wouldn't be any good at all. It got me thinking though, if I recognise that, if I can see that then why can't I do it? Why am I always looking back and looking at the negatives rather than looking forward and focusing on the positives? I watched a show called 'School of Hard Knocks', it features rugby legends Will Greenwood and my personal favourite Scott Quinnell, it's about people who've had a life of crime, bad upbringings and they all come together to form a rugby team, they have eight weeks to become a unit and it's filled with lots of ups and downs. Will, Scott and Chris Chudleigh are AMAZING people, the drive, the passion they have is inspiring. I remember watching a clip and it was Scott Quinnell talking about how you have to bring an aggressive mindset to rugby, it's a physical sport, if you watch it then you see it is. He was talking to the forwards about their mindset, he had the ball and physically charged over one of the coaches, he just picked the ball up and ran, after he bulldozed the coach he's heard to say "It's about a mindset, it's ABOUT THE MINDSET" and do you know something, he's absolutely fucking spot on, I still watch that clip of him, I watch many clips of him because I see someone with tremendous mental and physical strength, he's right. It is ALL about the mindset and that's what I need to work on, it is a fucking battle, I have to be ready for war at all times and if I don't have the right mindset I'm going to crumble, I'm going to get walked over and I'm going to lose, I'll get trampled. I need to get that ball and run over people, I can't stop until I reach that try line, whether it be boxing or rugby analogies the message is the same, I need the mindset and the fight to actually beat this, I need to score a try, I need to get a knockout, I need to win, if I can beat this then I'll consider my life worth living, I mean that's all that I want to do is live my life, that's it, that's all I ask, is that too much? I don't think that it is to be fair. I need to stop being so harsh on myself, I need to start being more chilled out and not so argumentative, I need to stop shouting at the TV when adverts come on that I hate, I need to take a step back and just enjoy life, whether it be playing pool, or golf, or the xBox or even the mega drive I need to have that switch that gets flicked off. For the first time in a while I'm looking forward to seeing my GP on Wednesday (12/11/2014) and admitting that although it's not been my best week I've wrote it all down and I'm facing my troubles head on, I'm not shirking it by hiding under the covers, I'm not hiding away and letting them get me. I'm now in a position where I want to tackle this and conquer it, whether I'll do it or not I don't know. I'm setting myself some really small goals just now and at the moment this focuses on seeing my GP week-to-week, I'm hopeful of then seeing myself to Christmas and then my birthday on January 15, at the moment though I'm focusing on Wednesday to Wednesday, day-to-day and hour by hour, small steps to start and then I can then start working on bigger ones. Short-term focus though is to stop being so hard on myself, give myself a break and look at any mistakes as just... mistakes and not massive failings. I'm viewing this too simply, a lot has happened and I feel my mind is waning again, it is 10/11/2014 at 15:01, it's been almost two days since my 'massive breakthrough', two days since I started to feel cleansed, started to feel good again and how do I feel now? I'll tell you how I feel, I feel like fucking shit again. I don't think it's a matter of looking 'at any mistakes as just... mistakes and not massive failings.' I don't think it's got anything to do with that, it's about that fucking mindset and my mindset is that I'm just not good enough for the people in my life, I'm not good enough for my family, I don't deserve being treated and cared for. I'm sitting here in my bed, curtains drawn with a cup of coffee constantly asking myself 'How am I feeling'? Is that a hard question? Should this be a question that causes your mind to speed up, is this a question that should flummox, confuse and agitate? Of course it's fucking not but when I'm asking myself that question I cannot fucking answer it, I can't physically tell myself let alone you how I feel today. I can't tell you how I FEEL, I can't physically tell myself how I AM FUCKING FEELING TODAY AND IT DRIVES ME ABSOLUTELY FUCKING CRAZY, I WANT TO GO OUTSIDE AND YELL, I WANT TO GO OUTSIDE AND FUCKING SHOUT AGAIN, I WANT TO RUN AWAY, I WANT TO CUT MYSELF, I WANT TO END THIS AGAIN, SUICIDE IS LOOKING LIKE MY ONE AND ONLY FUCKING OPTION AGAIN, IT'S NOT GETTING BETTER, IT'S GETTING WORSE, I'M FALLING, DETERIORATING, CRUMBLING, DISINTEGRATING, I COULD QUITE HAPPILY GO TO SLEEP JUST NOW AND NEVER WAKE UP, I COULD DO IT QUITE HAPPILY WITHOUT SAYING GOODBYE, I CAN'T EVEN TELL YOU OR ME HOW I AM FUCKING FEELLIIINNNGGG TTOOOOODDDAAAYYYY? DAVE, HOW DO YOU FUCKING FEEL TODAY? WHAT'S INSIDE OF YOU, WHAT... DO.. YOU.. FEEL?? The answer is that I don't know, I almost feel like my emotions are numbed, there's nothing, I'm empty, I have nothing inside me that I can share with you. All that seems to be there is this big flashing thought in the front of my mind that I'm not strong enough to beat this, how much longer can I hold out before the thought of taking my own life appeals to me more than living my life. I'm so calm though, it's like an icy-calmness, the kind of calmness that you only seem to feel when someone has scorned you, burned you really badly, it's the kind of calmness I fear because I know that it's going to change, it's going to morph into a massive motherfucking set of demons again, it's going to drain every single drop of mental strength that I have, there's a fight coming again and I need everyone, I can't talk to anyone, the only way I can find solace and comfort is writing it all down, I want to get every single person I love together and tell them, I want to sit them down and physically tell them that genuinely I believe their lives would be better off without me, my family would be better off without me and the world would be better off without me. Why do I continue to battle this when the feeling inside is that the war will be lost, what is the point of soldiering on when I feel like I'm going to succumb. Is the numbness wearing off? I've not taken my medication in three days, I don't want to take the medication, it doesn't do anything and I don't feel any different when I do take it. I'm beginning to doubt again, Saturday's exorcism was temporary, it was a lift but only a short one, I've woken up on this cold November Monday and as soon as I've woken up the demons have hit me with a sobering wake-up call: 'Morning Dave, remember how you're a loser, remember how long you've battled this, always remember for every good day you have I'll visit it back four-fold and twice as nasty, I'm ALWAYS going to be here, here in your mind, lurking.. always there ready to strike you when you think life is going to be great. Get up, get up Dave, take the meds, take them, go on, they'll make you better, you'll feel better. Better? HA! Of course you're not, I'm too strong for them, is that the best that you've got? Pfft, how about a drink Dave? Some alcohol would make you feel better, ooooo you have the house to yourself Dave, there's the balcony, should we go outside? It's nice outside, look ahead Dave, look at all you see, relaxed? Look down Dave, look down.. LOOOOkkkk DooowWWNnnn Dave, it takes one jump, it takes one single moment of courage, do you have it? Can we do it? You need sleep Dave, eternal sleep, do it. Come on, think of the misery, the hate, the hurt, the scars, open the scars, think of every single thing that you've done wrong in your life, I've scrambled all the good things you do so you can't see them, do you want to fight another day? Take me on, come on Dave, start fighting back'. I am, I am fighting back... By not doing it I'm... fighting. I feel weak, my eyes hurt, my head hurts but my mind doesn't, my mind gets stronger each day but I don't. I'm two seperate entities, I am body and mind, the mind controls all, the mind is the hub, the epicentre of my being, it's in control of me again, I had control for little over a day, it felt good, I like(d) being in control of my mind, I can see Wednesday, I can see my GP, I can talk to him, I won't hide, I can tell him, I can tell him that I'm not insane, I'm fighting. My eyes are fighting back, if I don't close my eyes I don't see the pain, with my eyes open it's blurred, I see the good things I do, I see myself as Dave, I see myself having laughs, I see my friends, I see Darren, Pamela, Claire Fullerton, Stuart McIlwain, Leigh Halliday, Jillian Graham, I see an army behind me, I have the strength and the will, I have a sword, forged with the love of hundreds of friends and it cuts through the darkness, I see everyone I've been fortunate enough to meet and get to know, I appreciate the time they've taken to get to know me, not only know me but understand me, they UNDERSTAND me, not only do they know me but they understand me, that's huge. I've let them in, they see me as I am, I don't have to act happy. If I can't look at them I don't have to, I'm having a bad day, they see that. I don't feel bad that I can't talk to them, I'm having a bad day, they see that. They've seen me through some pretty bleak times. I want to repay all my friends, I want a night out in Glasgow for my 33rd birthday, (what date was my birthday again?) I want to go out singing and getting drunk, oh wait, I read between the lines of that, fuck, no, no..... If I flip that I'm actually saying on my 33rd birthday I want to get drunk and go out singing, I can't go out on my 33rd birthday can I? I can't, 'check out', 'buy the farm' etc on my birthday? Can I? No, I don't want to. Am I insane, can I ask myself that? How am I feeling today, am I feeling insane? No, I don't think I am, I don't feel right though, I've been laughing and joking with Steve today playing games, I like it. I felt good. I've got light and music with me just now, I do feel good, it's the darkness I fear, when it gets dark they all come out to play, the darkness is where they breed, it's where they grow and expand. No... please, leave me alone, please? Please..?

I've never dug this deep before so I'm not really sure what I'm going to say, I still feel I can dig even deeper, I need to find the root of this before I go back to work, if I don't the cycle will start again, projected/estimated timeline below:

12/11/2014: See my GP, tell him I feel much better, I've thought about suicide but it's not as dominant, neglect to mention what I've written previously in the book and generally I'm doing better. I'm happier (I'm not)

13/11/2014: Put big massive update on Facebook that I'm better, I've beaten it yet again and no-one/nothing is going to stop me. (They are/it is)

17/11/2014: Return to work 25/12/2014: Christmas, see the family, life is good.

15/01/2015: Birthday, life is good, notice an increase in Facebook posts about drunkness, various topics and general attention-seeking .

March 2015: Decline nights out, cancel plans and have a few beers in the house instead

April 2015: Start getting angry at everyone and start to feel insecure about myself

May - July: Drink but don't admit I may have a problem

18 August: Drink and start to write things down September: Most likely break down and start crying at work. Maybe write a book? That may appear cynical but it does go in a cycle and that's my fault because I let it happen, I neglect my mental health, I neglect my physical health and by the time I decide to do something about it it's too late, they're there and I've left myself too much to do. My 'condition/illness' is something that I

feel comfortable discussing now but if I took better care of myself it wouldn't happen as much as it does, do you know one of the reasons why it does happen though? I'll tell you. I have no resolve, I have no willpower, I'm famous for it. I once swore blind that I was going to go vegetarian, it was 2009 and I'd decided this was the life for me, I had one 'albondigas salad' (Stuart McIlwain, LOL!) and I bet I didn't even last three days before I went back to eating meat. The amount of times I've said I'm going to stop drinking, I'm going to stop swearing, the amount of times I've just simply said I'm going to do something my friends are like 'Aye right Dave, sure.' Do you know something, they're right, when I worked in Glasgow all it would take to break me was someone to ask 'fancy a pint after work'? That was it, that is all it would take for me to go out in Glasgow and end up getting absolutely fuckin' steamin', I'd fall asleep on the train, end up in Stirling and end up phoning my Dad for a lift because I had no money, what a dick eh? I know he doesn't mind but it's not the point, I should be more respectful towards my Father, I'm sorry, I didn't mean to be a dick, it just.. comes natural to me. Thank god I'm not a smoker or do drugs.I would actually be dead by 35 and it wouldn't be my decision, my lungs would be tar-fucking black if I smoked and drugs I don't even want to think about. (I have three pints of Heineken and I'm pished, fuck knows what drugs would do to me, probably end up streaking through a police station and putting one of their hats on my willie. ('A'right officer, weh-hey I've got yir hat oan ma willie', woooooo, helicopter time!') Probably best I don't touch drugs eh? I'm actually quite strong willed when it comes to not touching drugs, basically because I know they'd well and truly fuck me right up. Reading that back it has a sense of irony, I am fucked up, I'm well and truly fucked up but drugs would amplify it, drugs would make me do it, I know that so I steer clear of them. I make my own head hurt, all that I've written is what goes on my head, no wonder my head hurts. It's weird though because although I've got all that going on there's a wee part of my head that churns out funny wee names, I giggle to myself, Steve giggles as well, we make each other giggle. For example our old dog that died Cassie, (fuck you Pottie) we named her 'The Baron' between ourselves, I don't know why, for the new pup Misha we nickname her 'The Great Van Gatso', don't ask, we don't know. Makes us fucking laugh though, imagine walking your dog and you've got to shout one of those names? I think I'd belly-laugh, I like belly-laughing, it doesn't happen as often as it should, it happened once with Pottie and it was in 2009, you know what 'Secret Santa' is eh? Well one of the chaps got Mr P a bottle of whisky in a rather nice looking box (he likes whisky, he's a refined chap.)

but there was a twist, in the box unbeknown to us was a bottle of vodka, (he HATES vodka) well that was it, we were in a restaurant and I lost control, I BURST out laughing, I couldn't stop laughing, I'm pretty sure I started banging on the table I was laughing that hard, I laughed for ages, I still laugh, I'm laughing now, it was soooo funny. To this day I've never been able to replicate THAT laugh. To this day I still see his face and the utter dejection that came across it. (Lolzer, kiss) Anyways, I think you get the point with that, it was one of the funniest moments I've ever seen and I will never ever forget it! Me and Steve do it a lot though, we're not brothers really, well.. we are but we get on so well, we just laugh about anything really, I feel like a much better person whenever I'm near him. He makes me feel human, he makes me feel good and he doesn't even know it, he's so mellow, chilled, laid-back and completely fucking lackadaisical, we couldn't be more opposite in terms of persona, I've seen him actually angry on a few occasions and it's scary, for him he sees me angry at everything, I shout at the fridge, I shout when I drop my keys, I shout when I bang my elbow off doors. I just... shout a lot. He's the one person that never leaves my mind, my Mum, Dad and all my lovely friends float out at some point but he's always there. I'm so proud of him, he's a worker, a grafter, he's a really genuine person and he makes my world so much better for being in it. I share the flat with him, I get the rent and he gets amenities, it's a good arrangement, it's a nice arrangement, I wouldn't share a flat with anyone else except him. The fact that he's just in the next room quell my thoughts of suicide. In 2011 I didn't have him with me, well I had him but I stayed on my own, with him in the house I can't drink, I can't have fizzy juice, remember what I said about resolve? Yea' without him I'd be drinking heavily again and I would be well and truly fucked. I'd be on the final level of Road Rash II with the best bike, one bar of 'bike health' and seven miles to go, the bike goes 180mph so yea', I'd be fucked. He makes the bike health full, he puts me in control and he makes me believe that I can finish the race. Saying goodbye to him would be the toughest thing I would ever do. I just.. don't think I could face it, I wouldn't want to see the look in his eyes, even when I was dead I'd still see it. I'd hate myself for ruining his life. Steve if you ever read this you mean the absolute world to me and without you I'd be dead, simple as that. I understand though for anyone to get to this point reading is an achievement, it's heavy going, it's not been easy for me to write, well actually it has. This all.. poured out without too much coaxing, I don't know if I'm insane, I don't know if I'll ever summon the power to beat this, I don't know if I'll get through this battle. If I do I want to meet people, I want to talk about it and I want there to be no barriers. I've never finished reading a book before let alone write one, when I first had this idea ten days ago I thought it was along the lines of stopping drinking or being a vegetarian, I thought I'd write one-hundred words and then just give...up, I'm a pro at giving up, I'm a pro at quitting as I've described, I've no willpower, I've no real desire but here I am, at my worst state and I'm choosing to write, I'm choosing to put this out there not just for my friends and family to see but the world. I don't feel any shame about anything I've written, I'm glad I swore, I'm glad that I got that all out of me, my head hurt after it and I was glad. I have held absolutely nothing back in this, I have reached way down inside of me and pulled some pretty nasty bile out, I've ripped some roots out and I've been able to share them with you. I've done something that I've never been able to do before and that's being completely 100% open. I'm glad I met Stephen Heggie and Stuart McIlwain on Friday, I'm happy I cried, I'm so proud of myself for saying I may not make it through this, they know that if I don't I gave it 100%, I'm giving it 100%, I want to beat this 100% and for you that read this I thank you 100%, this was a great outlet, it was something I'm glad that I've completed. It's an achievement. I'm going to close this off by just saying a few things if I may. I mean what I say when I say I want to beat this, I think I've got many things to offer society and an early death wouldn't do it justice. Although I feel different I feel like it's not a bad thing anymore and I need to be myself in society's eyes, in my own mind I have the confidence to be myself but I need to find it. Once I do I can start being the type of guy that I was born to me. Brilliant, diverse, funny, genuine, caring, honest, open. I want to go out with my friends again, I want to see Glasgow and enjoy all it has to offer, I want to wear bright colours, shave my head and have a massive beard, I want to wear glasses with no lenses, wear a million ties, get drunk and post drunken pictures on Facebook, I want to live and be happy living. I don't know who you are, that's a shame because I bet you're really cool, I want to let you know that there is hope however bad you feel, write a book, sing a song, talk to friends, talk to family, paint. There are ways to feel better, even when you're contemplating suicide. I'm still thinking about it but in the minutes, hours, days, weeks and months to come I hope to start seeing the good days, get some good music on (I've got 'stevie' by 'Kasabian' on, fucking belting tune, I can't tell you how much that's helped me open up.) Take care of yourself and take one day at a time. Whoever you are I love you. If you're in Glasgow let's grab a few pints, play pool and get drunk. If I don't make it then please remember that I gave it my all but in the end my demons were too strong for me, I gave in but not before I explored all options. Be seeing you.

February 2015 – May 2015

I fucking irritate myself, I truly mean that. I wish that I had an identity, a persona. Instead I adapt myself to the people around me, I'm a social chameleon and I don't fucking like it. I'm too scared to be myself around people, I'm too worried that I won't be everyone's friend and I'm scared that I say something that won't be in line with the company I find myself in at any particular time. I'm 33 and I'm still trying to find myself, I don't know what I think of myself and I just cannot seem to get going at all. So what's been happening since I last wrote, I now have no job, I'm back living with my parents as I have no flat and oh yea', I nearly committed suicide back in December, so yea', nothing has happened at all…. I am so fucking sick of my head, I'm hateful of the person I am and I'm hateful of my uncanny ability to not know what the fuck is going on inside of me. I don't think I'll ever be faulted on effort, I put so much in each and every single day and although things have been good lately a lot of that has been down to me and turning negatives into positives. Do you know something I'll say this before I start getting into this and it's the one thing

I feel I know about myself: I HATE society and I hate being forced to be a part of their fads, trends and fucking obsessions with music. I drink a lot but when I do it helps me to escape the mind-numbing humdrum of the daily grind. On reflection I think it would be better if I were to be cast adrift from society and left to drive myself insane. So it's been over three months since I wrote all of the above and I'm pleased to report that I am in a much better, stronger place now, at the time of writing that I was in such a bad place and to be honest I think I was a little bit raw from my attempted suicide on 28/12/2014. So before I start delving into things I'm going to go through a couple of things that's happened. At the time of writing it's 24/05/2015 and it's bang on 11am. Lots has happened since I last wrote and the majority has been great. So what's been happening in my life, well instead of being called Dave I've decided to take my father's name so I am now called Davy, I've managed to secure a really good job and I've decided to devote my life to being completely and utterly celibate, so yea', both me and my mind have been busy. I think I'll start with the celibacy thing, it just feels like the right place to begin things, it's the biggest decision I've made in my life up until this point and I'll explain the reasoning why, I didn't really touch on it in my previous book but then again at the time of my previous writings I really wasn't in a great place at all, infact who I am I kidding at the time of writing my last one I was close to death, I did state at the end I may not make it through this and at the end of December I tried to quit, I overdosed and I had made my peace with it. I had said my goodbyes and that was it. I took about 30 tablets, I can't remember the exact name of them but I remember the feeling of my chest tightening up almost immediately and me sitting on my bed ready to die. I text my brother saying goodbye and that I was sorry for putting him through this but enough was enough. The previous week I stood on the balcony of my top floor flat and nearly jumped, I was hospitalised twice in a week. I really came THAT close, I mean I actually attempted to take my own life, actually just writing this and thinking about it I 'm really grateful to all around me, I have an amazing support network and they got me through a phenomenally horrible time. Infact it wasn't just horrible for me it was horrible for everyone concerned. I never ever want to put my family through that again. I will never ever forget the look on their faces when I came to in hospital. So over the last five months I've been solely focused on building my mental strength, it's been a long road but I finally feel strong within myself again, I feel like I've always felt I should be. I feel confident, I feel strong and I feel ready to kick on. I'll be 100% honest, I genuinely don't think I give myself nearly enough credit for the amount of strength I have and the things I have actually achieved, I am way too harsh on myself and that's one of the many things that I have actually managed to banish. As this goes on and I start to delve deep inside me I'll try to take you with me and try to let you see what I see and feel what I feel. I'll try, I can't make any guarantees you'll see it but I'll do my absolute best. At points as well I'll be writing after having a few beers, with just the right amount it helps me open up a little bit more, I'll let you know when that happens as well, throughout this I will hopefully be able to fully delve and come out of this even stronger. Make no mistakes this is going to be hard for me. Everything that I write is going to present it's own obstacle or challenge. I don't want you thinking that me writing this is going to be a cakewalk. This is going to be fucking hard work because what I'm going to do is basically strip myself down, break myself open, expose myself at my weakest and then look to build myself back up, now that's territory I've been to before but not to the extent that I'm going to attempt in writing this book. The first one compared to this was easy because I was at my absolute lowest, the words came easy as the feelings were at my fingertips, this I think is going to be a lot tougher to write.

I'm not saying this just to be different and I'm certainly not saying it to make myself sound cool, I'm saying this because I genuinely believe it. My wiring is different to the majority of society's, it's something that I've always believed and I do think I feel more than the average person. I have a tremendous amount of empathy, it's at a point where I use it almost for 95% of conversations, I can't help it, when someone is speaking I almost always jump into an empathetic state of mind, it happens automatically like just getting up and washing my face or putting my pants and socks on at the start of my day, I mean it just happens. Now that doesn't sound normal to me, it's something that has always happened and I can't turn it off. I'm not saying it's a bad thing, I'm just saying I think it's different and it allows me straight away to 'feel' my way around a conversation more than an average person. I'd like to point out straight away I'm not saying I have a totally unique mindset, I'm trying to point out a number of different factors that all contribute to my struggles and battles with depression. I am way too much of a nice guy, I'm nice to the point where sometimes I actually want to punch myself in the face, yea' it sounds harsh but it's true, I bend over backwards for people and I always put other's needs before my own. Once again it's something I've always done. I over-think, I mean I really over-think, my head never switches off and this is something I touched on in great detail in my previous work. I don't think this helps, I really don't.. I would love nothing more than for my brain to switch off but I just don't have that capability. Plus a lot of the time I never really know what's going on inside my head and by that I mean I'm always unsure of what other people's perceptions are of me, this is a HUGE factor in my depressive state, this is the one thing that cripples me when I have my bad days and the reason for that is that this one thought, this one conundrum in my mind wears me down and I never stop thinking about it. I mean this is an actual obsession, touch wood that it's not been bad lately but when it strikes it causes me to (over) analyse every single thing I do. Some typical examples of this are: • Speaking: - Hmm, could I have made that better? - Was my tone inflection correct? - Was my emphasis right? - Oh fuck did they think I was a cheeky fucker there, oh shit.. - Why did I say that, she hates me now. - Fuck you Davy, you've blew it. • General: - Am I walking ok? - Do I look confident? - Don't look down. Don't look down, you need to look confident - Your music is too loud - Do the people on the train think this band is ok? - Am I dressed ok today? What if I'm not dressed well. I mean I don't know if any of that makes sense but that's a little bit of what I go through when I'm having a not so good day, I refuse to say bad day now because that just amplifies/increases the speed of my thoughts. I've learned a lot from my depression and I think I'm managing it better. On 97% of my days these thoughts don't even enter my head, I'm confident, personable, attentive and ready to attack whatever the day has instore for me, but on the 'not so good days' it's an achievement I'm actually able to get out of my bed and believe me, that is hard work on one of those days. It.. is... fucking.... awful.. *sad face* I don't know why I care so much about people's perceptions of me. I mean at the end of the day does it really matter? I mean really, DOES IT MATTER? The honest and direct answer is no, it really fucking doesn't. (You'll see my language really hasn't improved at all throughout this, honestly it's fine though, I think it makes it easier to get points across. I may be wrong but I can't be the judge of that. The truth is I like swearing, end of) All of the above (with the exception of swearing) I have really put a lot of effort into and I think now I've managed to eradicate a lot of the self-doubt and the panicking. It's still a work in progress but I think I'm doing ok. Infact no scrap that, I don't 'think I'm doing ok', I AM doing ok. No actually I'm doing well. I need to be more positive, I've been working on being more positive and it's definitely making a difference, plus for the first time in years I'm actually comfortable in my own skin, that makes a massive difference both psychologically and socially. I think this is the strongest I've ever felt, I actually feel really good within myself and that comes across. I'm not doubting myself as much, I'm not over-thinking as much and I think I am looking really good. I think I decided to practice celibacy at the wrong time. D'oh! That leads me on to another point. A lot of the time in my head things have always been 'wrong', whether they actually were wrong or if it was just a state of mind have yet to be proven, I contributed a lot to my own problems because I didn't manage my state of mind correctly. For example on a particularly stressful day at work I would deal with this by 'having a few drinks', now my definition of a few drinks differs. When I'm out with friends me going for a few drinks generally involves a night out, the standard term is to go out and have 'a few drinks', when I'd had a not so good day a few drinks meant I would go to the shop, buy six cans of beer, have them and do that over three to four days a week, so I wasn't just having a few beers, I had an alcohol problem and I was using a bad day as an excuse to drink, there is a massive difference between the two and to be honest I lead myself to drink a lot of the 'bad/not so good days'. I've always had a dependency on alcohol, at my worst it's really quite bad though. It's hard a lot of the time, I mean it really is, from the time I left 3 on 02/05/2014 and by the time I went off sick from my last employer so much had changed within me, I wasn't the same person and I think a lot

of it was to do with the fact that I didn't have that 'support network' in a

professional environment, before I could go into work, have a quiet day

and not talk to anyone and it went from that to going in every day and

hiding how I was feeling. People at 3 understood me and they knew I

would have a couple of days downtime then be back to my usual self

again. In my last job I didn't have that and I made the cataclysmic mistake

of hiding my depression, the end result being on 01/09/2014 I lost

control, I couldn't hide it anymore and I broke down, that was the start of

the worst ever period of my life and if I could do the whole thing again I

would do it so much different. Actually, one thing that definitely didn't

help was the fact that I pissed away a sizeable redundancy in the space of

three months. I would tell you just how much I pissed away but you'd

never look at me the same again. Just before I continue here's a quick

question. What do you think I blew my redundancy on? Was it: a) A

holiday b) Strippers c) Booze Yip you're right, I did manage to blow a lot of

my money on nights out because I was 'happy', yea' I wasn't happy, I was

an alcoholic with basically a large amount of tokens, looking back on it I

did not handle the transition well. Thankfully though I am now in a place

where I can look at it, acknowledge it and move on whereas before I would look at it, analyse it, overanalyse it, think about it, agonize about it

and then worry about it. Having a much sharper, clearer state of mind

helps me to review things rather than over-analyse things, generally as

well I am now looking forward rather than living in my past, it helps,

believe me. Even though that happened a while ago it still hurts a lot, at

the start of this remember I said this wasn't going to be easy for me? Yea'

that stings a bit going back over it and not just for what I've written. See I

was off from the start of September and I didn't handle my time off well

either. Although I had a really fragile state of mind I don't think I

approached it the right way. See the problem I had was that I was alone a

lot and the reason for that was because some days I just couldn't face

anyone, now that in itself was fine but I spent a lot of my days just

wandering around the house in my pyjamas and then just playing xBox, I

didn't really adventure out, I shut the curtains and I basically barricaded

myself inside my house, I also didn't wash my face for about three

months, infact I didn't wash my face from 01/09/2014 until 24/11/2014.

Now under normal circumstances I would be thinking the same as you, I'd

be like 'eww, three months without washing your face, gros'. Yea' it

would have been but when you suffer you don't see it like that. What did I

have to wash my face for? I wasn't seeing anyone, I wasn't doing anything. All I would do is get up in the morning, have breakfast and then put the xBox on, that is all that I would do and that went on for months. I wandered from room-to-room thinking what am I doing, I found it hard to see my parents because I couldn't let them know how I was feeling, I struggled to talk to my friends, I couldn't. What would I say? I didn't know what to say to them. I didn't even know what was going on in my own head for fuck sake. It took all my effort to get up and out of bed, that in itself was a huge achievement, some days I would even open the curtains but that was on a REALLY good day, I mean that was on a REALLY GOOD DAY, they didn't come along often though. Looking back on it I actually spent a lot of time living like a recluse, I didn't particularly enjoy it but well, it happened and I can't really change it. See this is what makes it hard for me to talk to anyone when I don't feel right within myself, I can convey this all to you and to be honest I don't know what you're thinking, I doubt I'll ever know what you're thinking. All I want to get across really is the fact that as long as I live I will always be battling this. I am always going to be trying to conquer this and I'm accepting that this is my life. I don't think that I would want it any other way to be honest and I'm going to explain why I wouldn't want to be like anyone else: I find a lot of life boring, this socialistic ideal of the wife and two kids by the time you're in your thirties just pisses me off. Getting the nice suburban house that everyone else in your street has just doesn't appeal to me. Doing the garden on your day off and taking the kids to the park just doesn't cut it for me and besides, I've got more than enough to manage on my own never mind if you throw in a wedding, a wife and the thought of me being a father, that just flat terrifies me. I'm quite happy being on my own but then I know if I'm on my own I can make my own timetable, obviously now I'm back in work I'm referring to managing my time out of work. How would I manage my mental state with having a wife and kids, how would I get across to them that I needed some time on my own, what would I do if I got one of THOSE days where I physically couldn't talk to anyone? One of those days where I have to be on my own and there's nothing I could do? One of THOSE days where I end up wandering around Falkirk or Glasgow aimlessly with the simple intention of just... killing time? I don't think I could do it, would the wife understand? What about the kids? How would I explain that 'Dad just needs some time on his own', this can happen for days at a time, this doesn't limit itself to one day, I mean could I do that? I don't see myself being able to manage that. And this brings me back to the point I made at the start of this chapter, it's all about wiring, we're all wired different but we share some of the same components, I think I share a lot of the same wiring but there's just that odd switch or two that causes my thinking and my being to be a little deeper than your average joe. Then again though are my thoughts and my fears different than anyone else's? Is it maybe just all in my head and I am actually normal? I just perceive myself to be different in the hope it distinguishes me just that little bit from everyone else? Or am I actually different in terms of the waves of thoughts that overcome me and threaten to drown me from time-to-time. I genuinely don't know, if I did I probably wouldn't be taking this on and I would probably be doing a regular Sunday job like mowing the garden or painting the fence. There has to be something in the way I feel, I mean there just has to be. I don't think the things I experience/have experienced are normal. I've managed this(poorly at times) for over fifteen years now, something happened when I was eighteen that triggered this and I don't know what. I mean around that time I first started listening to a lot of Nirvana rather than the mainstream pop that I'd grew up with. Did I maybe hear a lyric that started me thinking, was there something in me that changed? Did I have a chemical imbalance that peaked that year, I don't know regrettably but I'd love to go back and see what I was like back then. Infact that's something I think about a lot, going back to the year 2000 and living through that year to see what kind of things I was thinking and doing. Did something happen that's been hidden away in the back of my memory or could it be there is just no explanation, maybe it just.. happened and I didn't realise it. All I know is I'll never find out unless I happen to invent something that allows me to go back and honestly would I do it if I had the chance? No, I probably wouldn't because I would most likely fuck myself up, that would be weird going back and being inside your own head all those years ago. Yea', I think it's best if that's just left in the past. Maybe I'm looking at this in too complex a fashion, maybe there's a way to just simplify all that's in my head rather than getting the world's biggest blackboard and psycho-analyse every single thought that goes through my head. Like rather than me over-thinking and stressing why could I not just let what's happened live in the past and just look to my future. I mean that's what I have been doing since February and the results are pretty good. I think it's a good thing to acknowledge your past but it's definitely not good to try to live in it, I mean that just screws with your head, it certainly did with mines anyways. I think about death a lot, once again it's just one of those things that's always been there. I don't think of it in terms of like 'I want to die' but I often wonder what actually happens when death comes. I mean do you get the white light and the big flashback, do you get to look down on people and continue to look over your loved ones after you're gone or do you get to come back and do some really cool haunting. I would LOVE to do that, people that I didn't like and I would just fuck with their chi, like when they're in a bath and I would flicker the light, or put some random bread in their toaster. OR I would just move all of their stuff about and drive them nuts. I totally want to be a ghost when I die, I wouldn't be like your stereotypical ghost, I'd be a 'cerebrally talented' ghost, I would so fuck with your head. But on a serious note what happens when you die, I mean it's one of those things that's really down to your own interpretation I guess, now I'm not going to get into religious beliefs here because quite frankly I often find these discussions/debates rather tedious. I've just often wondered what happens after you go, it's just one of those things that runs round my head.

Ugh, I dreaded this bit but if I get it out now then I won't need to cover it later. I've never really been in a meaningful relationship, the previous partners I've had have all been ok but I don't think I've ever felt the whole love thing. Since the age of eighteen I've had maybe three/four girlfriends and to be honest it's just never really worked. I mean I know a lot of pretty girls, I'm definitely lucky that way and yea' I fancy a few of them but I know in my heart of hearts me and relationships would never really work. - I lack confidence - My mental state That's pretty much it, I mean the relationships I've been in have all broken down because of me, I either just lost interest and in one I actually cheated on my partner, I'm not proud of that. I think I'm just one of those guys who is going to be better off on his own, that was the main reason for my decision a few weeks ago to practice celibacy, the last time I had sex was January 2013 and to be honest I don't miss it. I mean yea' it's nice and if you get the right partner it can be great but I'm not really bothered. I mean I'm really not. I don't have the confidence or the desire needed for a relationship. By deciding to become celibate I've taken a lot of the pressure off of me because I am no longer dressing or acting to try to attract members of the opposite sex, that was one of the big worries in my mind, because I'm naturally insecure I would spend ages in the morning trying on lots of different combinations and instead of picking something I was comfortable in I was picking clothing to try to make myself more appealing to the females I worked/commuted with. Now, I don't think I'm a bad looking guy, don't get me wrong I'm never going to win Mr Universe or appear in a 'Greatest Hunks of All Time' calendar but I have a lot going for me. I'm not going to list what I feel are my strengths because frankly I've a lot but 99% of the time I look nice and I smell nice. I wear decent clothing and generally I feel great. The problem I had was that I was trying to attract just anyone, I get attracted to girls quite easy and to all different shapes and sizes, personally I prefer curves but that's my own personal preference. The problem I had was when I first met a girl whether it was in work or on a night out my first thought (if I was attracted to them) was 'Hmm, I wonder if they're single', now that I know for a fact is the complete wrong way to look at someone because 90% of time I'm going to be disappointed as I know they've got a partner, the other 10% would be me just thinking to myself 'Should I ask them out' or 'I wonder if they like me'. Now when I look back on that I realise my mistake and I now no longer do that. When I first meet someone now I just act like myself, also now that I'm not looking for anyone I know that takes a lot of the pressure off because I am comfortable in my own skin and not trying so hard to impress. Women can tell when you're doing that, women know a lot. At the same time though I mean I don't think I've ever really been that bothered though, I mean yea' there were times when I was looking for a relationship but I was always 'just looking', I never really went out on a lot of dates, I guess that's just the way it happened. To be honest there's too much in my mind I've got to control, that's why I think it's always been best that I'm single and besides, for the first time in a long while I'm now in a place where I am truly happy within myself, if I was to look at being with someone, now would be the time to start looking. I mean I still look at women in a normal way, I still get attracted to them and I still think normally, my celibacy hasn't changed the way I look at them. I'm at a point in my life where I want to start achieving and the new job that I started on 05/05/2015 is definitely the place where I want to be. I need to start looking at goals I want to set, although I'm only thirty-three I'm at a point in my life and my career to really start doing something wonderful. The key thing for me is going to be keeping on top of my mind and ensuring that if there is something wrong I speak to someone about it. I know exactly who to speak to as well should something go wrong. The relationships I truly treasure are my family and friends, I have had and am still having the privilege of meeting some truly fantastic people, now I only started my new job three weeks ago and I went out on Friday with them and we got absolutely steamin' drunk, I mean we got absolutely shit-faced and legless and this is only after three weeks. I am really lucky in the fact that whatever job I am in I always get a really good training group that I always end up making great friends with, it's the same in any job that I've had I always end up meeting great people and they all mean the world to me. I don't know how I always end up with this happening but I don't care, I hope to know these people for the rest of my life, although I have my struggles and my ups/downs I know these people are going to be there for me, that in itself gives me a lot of strength, I value friendship higher than I value anything else. I could never be one of those people with lots of money with hundreds upon thousands of fake friends. I would rather live my life and have the people I have over thousands of hangers-on who only hang around with me for money. Incidentally, to any of my friends reading this if you are hanging around with me for money I'm afraid I don't have much, sorry! (Laugh out loud) In all seriousness I depend on my friends and family as without them I'm nothing. Without them I have nothing to strive for, nothing to better myself for, I don't have any reason to make myself live for without them. Because I do have them though I can get up in the morning and know I've got to give whatever I do 100%, whether that be the current training I'm doing for my new job, whether it be playing snooker or whether it be going on a night out with the various social circles I have. One thing is for certain, they will always continue to motivate me to be better so to all of you guys I'm lucky to know, thank you from the bottom of my heart. You mean so much to me and you continue to give me strength. See that to me means one million times more to me than being in a relationship. I don't care much for them but I will always care for my friends. I know that they're always there for me and I'm always there for them. Friendship means more to me than anything and I wouldn't trade the people I had for all the money in the world. That's what made the period from September 2014 until December 2014 the worst of my life, I couldn't see them, I couldn't be with them and most importantly I couldn't talk to them, I couldn't talk to anyone for four months and it almost ended up with me losing my life, I can't even say that I'm sorry because the reasons for dying outweighed the reasons I wanted to live. It was a bloody, mentally draining battle that I fought so hard and so long for and it had won. That's the thing with depression, that's what people can't see, it's a war within the mind and although on the outside I looked fine, internally I was anything but. At the time of writing six months ago I thought I was coming out of it, I genuinely felt that I was making really good progress and in a month or so I'd be back to work, as it turned out I had absolutely no idea just what was going to transpire over the next six to eight weeks. I use social media a lot, well I use Facebook a lot, I used that as a means to update people around me how things were progressing and I think I used it quite well. It is oh so easy though to lie though, not just on social media but by texting as well. It's easy to stick a smiley face on the end of a post or a message and people can think 'oh he's fine, look he's smiling'. The truth is though that it's dead easy to do that and to fool people, if I could live that period of my life again I would do things differently. I didn't want people worrying, I felt as if my illness was taking up their time, I felt guilty, I felt as if I should just deal with this myself, other people have their own worries you know Davy. Infact, Davy... why are you doing this? Deal with this yourself because people have stuff going on too. Davy, ok? You deal with this, this is your responsibility, no-one elses.. ok?' That's what it was like, that's what was going on inside my head, I couldn't control it, I couldn't stop it and I couldn't change it. That done fuck all for my mood, infact I'd go as far as to say it put me back so much. See that was the other problem, I should never have been on social media with my mindset, I was of a very, VERY fragile mindset, now social media at the best of times is a mindfuck, never mind when you're battling depression and suicidal thoughts. I should have come off of it and ignored it, I didn't and I ended up fucking my mind up just that little bit more. Most commonly thought words from September - December - Useless - Needy - Suicide - Mindset - Mindfuck - Trying - Heavy - Not today A lot of that was hard for me to take. Depression is a pattern that's very hard to break. What is it like, it's like being in a moshpit, the other side is where you need to get to and to get there you've got to get through everyone there. They're the barrier and you've got to try and push through them. A lot of the time I couldn't even take a step, I thought about it and then went back to bed, this went on for months, I would actually lose track of days because every day just rolled into one another. (This is getting hard again) I kept getting up and I kept having my breakfast, hoping that one day I would have a sort of 'Eureka!' type moment, regreattably it didn't happen. It was hard going though, I know to a lot of people being off work because of 'depression' would seem like a sort of free pass to just… lounge about but it really wasn't. Every night I'd go to my bed so tired because all I would do all day is think, I got so fucking tired of thinking, I mean I really did because it was all I would do, god I got so fucking bored of it. Why was I thinking? Thinking never resolved anything because all I would fucking think about was my fucking past. Nothing good came from that, I would take my anti-depressant, have my breakfast and then go back to sleep. I would think, I would think, I would think…. (I got soooo tired of thinking, everything was just mush, everything got clumped together and would manifest itself as this big cycle, it would NEVER stop, it never gave me peace, I couldn't even lie in the bath without thinking, it never, ever stopped…….) By the end of it and when I was sitting with the pills in my hand I had thought myself quite literally to death, by the time I got there I was actually relieved, I was actually thinking 'Thank fuck, now I won't have to think anymore', that's what that done to me, over four months it had eroded everything inside me to dust and all I could think about was death, I mean what the fuck, I control my mind, my mind doesn't control me, I mean surely that's the way it should be right? Wrong. That for me was the battle right there, that key thought was the difference between my winning and losing. I fucking knew that if I could control my mind, I would win and if it controlled me, I lost, up until December my mind definitely controlled me and that's why I actually lost, just because I'm still here doesn't mean I won. I suffered a painful defeat and if it wasn't for my brother reacting and phoning 999 I wouldn't be here, I would have died. So yes, I did suffer a defeat but in the minutes, hours and days to follow after that I started to focus on beating this again. Was it easy to do so? No, absolutely not but trying to take my life and failing gave me a reason to start trying to defeat it again. I'd been to that place and I dared to set my feet over the edge, I made peace with myself and decided that life was for me again, this was it, I was going to give this my all and try to be the type of person I knew I could be. The type of person I had always dreamed about being but had never had the balls to actually be. So I tried to return to work one week after attempting suicide. My work quite rightly turned me away, regardless of how positive I felt there was no way I was ready to return, the thought was there and my intentions were good but no way was that my next move, I'm grateful to my employer throughout this whole time, they were amazing. Once again, another example of me being surrounded by excellent people. My support network is amazing. Unfortunately both myself and my employer both decided that we should part company, it was however the right thing to do as we both agreed that I needed to take some time to focus on my rehabilitation, it was correct and I'm glad that I did take that time, it gave me a period of time to kick-start my recovery and start to build up my mental strength.

I've never felt as if me and my mind were one entity, I've just always felt that either I've controlled it or more often than not it has controlled me. A lot of the times I think I could have controlled it but I think I've let it slip. I've never really been one for dealing with drama, some people have way too much it going on in their lives and personally I can just do without it. I'm actually a really simple being. All I really want in life is to have a decent job, a nice house, a games console and a few beers, seriously if I could have that then I will actually be contented. I know a lot of people are focused by money and unfortunately in these times it's hard to come by. I wouldn't say money isn't a priority, it is but it's not my ultimate end game. After everything I've been through and everything I've overcome it's time I got back to basics. I need to start looking at things that make me happy, a few of them include: - Watching/playing snooker - Playing xBox/Mega Drive - Listening to music, going to gigs - Walking the dog - Spend time with the family I mean realistically that's all my heart yearns for, I really don't want a lot out of life. If I had lots of money I'd be dead by the time I was forty. I wouldn't be good with a lot of money, it's a good thing I'm not really talented, if I was in the public eye I'd be an absolute fucking nightmare. I think about a lot of things, for example I hate how the UK has this massive 'celebrity culture', to be honest I couldn't give two fucks who wins Big Brother, who wins X-Factor, what retard 'wins' Geordie Shore and who eats the most bugs in 'I'm A Celebrity', is it news worthy? No. Do I give a fuck? No. I just don't see why we get so bothered about a group of halfwits trying to out ego each other. I shouldn't really read the papers or watch TV, it just has a tendency to get my blood boiling but I digress, it's probably better if I leave that behind or things will get ugly really quickly. Anyways, moving on. So I've never had difficulty relating to others but I have had difficulty with relating others to me. I tried for some years to let people in and see what I was seeing but I could never manage it. I think in a way that I never really wanted people to get it so I could retain some form of individuality and uniqueness. Now though I just don't see that as the best way to go, I've got a life to live. I've got a life that I tried to throw away five months ago. I want to try to help people that feel the same as me, people who suffer, struggle and have to fight to survive. If that means tearing myself down and re-building myself then so be it. For the first time in my life I've regained full control of my mind and I want to use that strength to help other people. I wouldn't go as far as to say it's my calling, that would be an incredibly pretentious thing to say, I've chosen to no longer hide behind my feelings and I want to share them with people. I have lived way too long in silence and in fear and to be honest I'm not going to stand for it anymore. Whenever I look back to my past I've always had a sense of being ashamed but I don't see why I should be? I mean why should I be ashamed or disappointed at something a lot of us go through? Why have I allowed myself to in some way feel inadequate when really I should be proud of all that I have achieved. This is exactly the way that I'm going to approach things and this is the way I've been thinking for the last two - three months, I've started to appreciate that the way that I feel isn't unique to me, it's something that a lot of people suffer from and I'm tired of the stigma that surrounds it. Mental health issues are just as important as physical health issues, just because you can't see a problem doesn't make it any less important. I felt very conscious about my problems and only a handful of people really knew what I had to endure. Now I'm not saying I'm going to be shouting things from the rooftops when I'm not well but I'm going to speak to someone about it. Rather than me sitting suffering in silence I'm going to talk about my issues and tackle it head on. A lot of people have that fear and believe me when I tell you it really isn't nice, it's a fucking horrible place to be and I wouldn't wish it on anyone. For the first time in my life I've now got the strength to talk about and tackle any issues that I have. Depression is a taxing illness and if we can talk about it more, we can help to break down the walls that's put up. That being said though I know it's not easy. I went for hours, even days at a time in a state of numbness. I didn't want to go out, I didn't want to stay in. I wanted to be with my family, I wanted to be on my own. I could never settle, I didn't sleep well, I didn't eat well and I didn't really take care of myself. Once again though it wasn't through lack of effort, it was just some days were hard. The strangest thing was though although I neglected myself the house was kept spotless. I done the washing when it needed done, I always made sure that dusting, hovering, bleaching was done. I tidied the livingroom, changed my bedding and made sure everything was clean, so I could look after the house but then I struggled to maintain myself. I think more often than not it was out of sheer boredom, I had the worst thing that someone of my mindset could have... a lot of time. I wasn't really seeing anyone so I had lots of time to myself and that was hard. There were times I was close to crying, there were days where I would sit on the couch and just look out the window, I wouldn't really do anything else, I'd just... sit. I wouldn't eat for hours, there were days I didn't eat. There was a time where I wore the same pyjamas for five days, I didn't have a bath, I didn't do anything. I just sat there, I sat there and I just... looked out of the window. That's all I done, it was all my mind would allow me to do and I could do absolutely nothing about it. I was helpless, trapped in my own head. There were no physical limitations, there was nothing to actually stop me from doing something but my mind would NOT allow me to do anything. As I'm getting into this I'm beginning to understand myself just what I'm saying, as I'm looking back it wasn't a state of mind. I was imprisoned within my mind, the tablets didn't do anything so I was basically trapped. Now you take that over a period of months, not just one or two days, this was every day I had to fight this off, I had to summon strength day after day to fight this, I fought so hard for so long and in the end I gave up. I can't sit here and say this'll never happen again, I wouldn't be so foolish or so arrogant to say that. What I need to do daily is to control what goes on inside of my head. That alone won't keep the demons out but it gives me a better chance of managing them, I don't think this is something that I'm ever going to defeat, it's something that I will always need to keep an eye on though. I know when things aren't right, I know what the warning signs are and from now on I'm damn sure if I see any of them they'll be heeded. It's like I'm being told 'you're not feeling right', what happens is: - A few days before I'll be completely hyperactive - Then I'll want to 'have a few drinks' - Then I'll start drinking excessively - Then I'll start listening to softer music i.e. Kelly Clarkson, Mazzy Star - Then I'll feel like shit and not want to talk to anyone. Normally I heed these warning signs and have a few days to myself, the problem was in my last job no-one knew I struggled with depression. Now I put this 100% on myself as I never said to anyone this was the case, when I started to have my struggles listed above I ignored them and carried on as normal and this links back to what I was saying about stigma. I was so scared to mention that I had mental health issues that I made myself really bad before I spoke up. I got to a point where I could no longer cope and I got myself in all sorts of trouble. I never ever want to go through that again, if I had just spoken to someone at the start when I began to feel bad then it could have quite easily meant I could have managed my situation better. I would urge anyone reading this if you don't feel right then talk to someone. Please talk to someone, anyone. Me not talking to someone very nearly cost me my life, I came perilously close, way too close. Now what I've said above may look like I'm blaming myself, I'm not. I'm saying I was scared to talk to someone about what was going inside of me, a mistake that I'll never make again. There's a lot going on inside me most of the time, I'm not very good at relaxing or doing nothing. I've always got to be doing something which I don't think helps. One thing I'm definitely looking at doing this year is relaxing more. So things like taking more baths, playing more snooker and get out more with the dog. I think that's something I have definitely neglected over the years and it definitely doesn't do me any favours, over the last few months I've been getting better at it and now that I've started work I've put in some groundwork into a work/life balance. I think that's going to be really important for the months and years ahead. Before my problem was that I would always take my work day home with me and vice versa, I never had clear boundaries and I suffered for it. Now I'm not saying I'm going to get this right 100% of the time but if I can get it working for me this will help with me keeping control of my mind and as I've stated

earlier, this is really important for me. I don't know why I've never really

been able to relax, it's just something that I've always sucked at, I'm

always 'on tilt' it seems, like always on edge, tight, rigid. Once again things

that do not help when trying to stay in control of my emotions. My life

isn't easy, now I'm not saying that so I can illicit tonnes of sympathy or get

a big hug but it's really not easy. I feel passionately about a lot of things

and they seem to hit me harder than what they hit the average person.

For example I can't read or watch anything to do with animal cruelty, that

just reduces me to tears instantly. I feel as if somehow my perception to

things like that has a heightened level of sensitivity, it reduces me to

rubble on the spot, especially if it contains anything to do with dogs, I love

dogs unconditionally and any sort of cruelty towards them makes me

want to find the perpetrator and rip their testicles out through their

mouth. I apologise for the super graphic nature of that but I feel very very

strongly about matters like that. You really don't want to get me started

on what I would do to people found guilty of animal cruelty. I'd make Jack

Bauer look like a pussy. With that in mind I'll move on. So you'll

remember I said I've never felt that me and my mind were one single

entity, I do genuinely feel that they are two separate components and my fight is going to be to get them working as one, I've never really felt that we work together, I always feel that me and my mind are fractured, I feel there's something that doesn't quite match up. Like I always feel that we're at odds and I'm always fighting for control. Maybe I over-think it too much, maybe I don't think about it enough? I actually don't know to be honest, it's a struggle and it's a pretty big drain on my mental resources, it takes up so much of my time and it's tiring. It affects my day-to-day workings, it affects my social interaction, it limits what I can and can't do and most importantly and critically of all it plagues my sleep. When I'm not in control of my mind I don't sleep, I just.. don't. it doesn't matter what I do I just will not fall asleep until about 3am and if I'm up at 6am then I don't need to paint you a picture of what the next day is like. This is why I'm hammering home the point of me being control of my mind, not my mind being in control of me. If I can keep doing what I'm doing and I'm in control I can shape my own future. I'm working so hard to be all I can be and it's imperative that I completely manage my emotions and continue to keep on top of things, I've worked too hard to make it to thirty-three years old, I need to hammer this home. So what have I been doing, well: - I'm not worrying as much - I'm not drinking as much - I'm not over-thinking as much - I've been relaxing more - I'm learning to be comfortable in my own skin - I'm getting better at switching off. All of those things combined make a massive difference, if I don't worry I don't stress, when I don't stress I don't drink, when I don't drink I relax more and when I relax more I tend to find I sleep better. Now that may sound like I'm stating the fucking obvious, I'm not, the way I look at it is all these small things combined equate to a huge difference in the way my life works. Each of those statements above are small parts which are part of a plan I put in place nearly six months ago, it's taken a lot of time and effort but it's something that was necessary to stop myself suffering. I'm not saying that for the rest of my life if I work to these principles I'll never suffer from depression but in terms of managing my thoughts and the cycles depression brings this has definitely been a keeper. I used to be really selfconscious, like I got up in the morning and I would scrutinise everything, I hated how I looked in the mirror, I didn't like my face and I could never find anything to wear. Now bear in mind this was all before I'd even left the fucking house so automatically I was behind, because I got up, lumbered to the bathroom, picked faults in everything I could see I was already behind, I had already said to myself 'I'm a loser', 'I suck', I had basically admitted defeat before my day had begun. I hated it but I couldn't stop it, I tried to see the positives but I just couldn't. Well, fuck that. I do not want to live the rest of my life like that, I'll be damned if I'm going to live the rest of my days with a frown on my face and wallowing in selfdoubt. That is no existence for me, yea' there's some days I'll get up and I don't look my best but I take that on the chin and just get on with it. 99.9% of days I get up, shave my head with a razor, take a good look in the mirror and I know that I am going to boss the day. I want to start like a winner. Because then if I start like a winner I stride on my walk to the train station, I walk confidently into work and then I'm already ahead of the game. It's about the mindset, I'm working on a permanent change of my mindset, it might take me six months, it might take me sixty years, all I know though is if I focus on the positives rather than my negatives I'll have a better chance of beating this and living a fulfilling and meaningful life, that's the plan anyways, whether it works out like that time will undoubtedly tell. When I look at the person I was back in December and the person that I am now it's like night and day, I'm so much more confident now and although I'm looking forward I find it rewarding to just take a glance back to the person that I was. Six months ago I was a shell of my former self, I looked ill, I was ill. I hid behind a pair of yellow sunglasses I didn't want other people looking at me, I wanted to feel invisible, human contact and interaction scared the hell out of me. The only time I would actually feel comfortable is when I spoke to my doctor every Wednesday, I genuinely looked forward to that as it meant I had gone another week without suicide, I'd made it another week and I had fought hard another week. Aside from that I never really felt comfortable being around anyone, my parents, my friends and even my brother who I shared a house with. I didn't feel as if I was worth anything, I felt miserable, poisioned, I felt as if I was insignificant, low, I felt as if I was nothing. I didn't feel as if I was worthy of anyone else's time, my conversation was a waste of my breath and I was a waste of their time. When I talked to professionals it felt as if I was making it up, I was being melodramatic and a hypochondriac, I genuinely felt that I myself was worth absolutely fucking nothing, it was a period of my life where I would quite happily have upped sticks, left and not said a fucking word to anyone. It was horrific.

I don't class myself as a good person, I have a niece and a nephew that I never see, it's not that I don't want to see them it's just I don't see myself as a positive influence as an uncle, plus my fear of children doesn't help my cause either... Seriously I have a huge fear of children, the farther I'm away from them the better, they give me the utter fear. Remember Rodney (Nicholas Lyndhurst) from Only Fools & Horses and his fear of

Damien? Yea', that pretty much encapsulates me. There are three things that I am utterly terrified of, in no specific order they are: - Children - Wasps - Spiders These are three things that give me the utter and absolute fear, there are probably one hundred things I would do before I ever had to be near any of the above. I just hope that my niece, nephew, (big) brother and wife understand I don't take any part in their life because I'm scared of children, I don't feel I have anything in common with them and my obvious battles mentally. I don't know if that makes me a bad person, I just hope that they understand that there are reasons for my absence. So at the moment I stay with my folks, I did stay in a really nice flat but due to my (little) brother moving in with his girlfriend in January and my work situation I had no choice but to move back in with the folks, it's fine, I love my parents but I don't like the person that I am when I'm here. My mood is very changeable and I don't like not being able to help/contribute with washing/ironing/tidying etc. My Mum has those covered but then again she always has done. I really don't like the person that I am and I feel that my folks are far too nice to me. I am looking to get my own place in Glasgow but this'll be after a few months when I've had time to bed myself into this job. At the age of thirtythree I just keep thinking that I should be doing better. I have very high-standards for myself, I always have done and I think that I always will do. It's just the way I am, I have an extraordinary high drive and I know no other way. I want to achieve in life, in that respect I class myself like other people. I take my life very seriously, now that's not an obvious statement as much as it looks like one. I think a lot about where I want to be in five years, I think about my career, I think about what's going to happen when my parents eventually go, I think about a lot, it may not look it at times but I'm very good at looking like I'm thinking of nothing when infact I'm thinking about everything. I always think about everything, it's a blessing and a curse in equal measures, some days I use it to plan ahead and sometimes I think myself to death with 'what if's' and 'buts', it depends on what mindset I'm in, some days it's really hard going, this is why I'm trying to just slow things down a little bit, my mind tends to race and I can get carried away. That needs to stop. Also, I don't know if it's such a good thing that I manage to be able to think really deeply when I don't look as if I am, it runs along similar lines to my ability to be able to hide how I'm really feeling, let's be honest that didn't really work out too well last time when I was with my previous employer so maybe I should look at dropping that. I think I should treat a 'not so good day' exactly as that, then at least I'll know I'm not forcing smiles or making myself worse. Does that make sense? To me it does but I don't know if it does to you. I'm trying here! So going back to my niece and my nephew, I think I'm doing the right thing but it doesn't feel as if I am? Now that statement isn't deliberate, it's an example of many things in my head where I think one thing but I feel another, I think it would be best for all concerned if I stay out of their lives and as I eluded to earlier it's not a selfish thing, I want to see them grow up and make successes of their selves, I just don't think that me being in their lives is going to be good for me or them, I may be wrong but I don't think I am. For once I'm going to trust my gut and go with the thing that feels right. I just hope one day they understand my reasoning and my logic behind this decision. Although I try I find it very hard to like the person that I am, I look at other people and I wish I was them, I look at smart people, funny people, people that can dance, people that invent things, people that seem to just find a way to get through life. I'm quite envious of other people, I wouldn't go as far to say jealous because I'm really not the jealous type. I just can't seem to settle on the person that I am, I've tried different looks, tried having a beard and being clean shaven, I really have trouble being myself, I can't settle on something that I'm happy with, my appearance is really important to me because if I'm not happy with how I look there's a good chance that I won't be happy with myself. If I'm not happy with myself then I'm not going to be happy mentally and if I'm not happy mentally then... well, you kind of know how that is going to pan out, for myself it really is not going to go well. I've been there and it's not a pretty place to be. Do you know what I sometimes do? I don't know if I should even share this but I'm going to anyway, I sometimes imagine that one of my friends has access to my mind, it happens sometimes when I'm in work, sometimes when I'm playing snooker, it happens even when I'm just lying in bed. I imagine they've got access to my mind, like when someone from IT takes control of your computer and they can see what you see? That's what I imagine, I think how I normally think but only someone else has eyes and they can see exactly what I'm thinking. That's quite weird eh? I don't know what triggers it, I've tried so hard to work it out but I've just not been able to work out quite why I think that. The thing is that it seems to re-focus me, it tends to weed out the bad thoughts and channel the good but as you'd expect that's only a temporary state, it never lasts longer than ten to fifteen minutes, fuck knows how that started, I don't know if I believe it or not but I think the reason that I do it is to try to let people in, even if it's not real it's almost like I'm trying to open myself up. Strange. Another thing that I do which I don't like is I tried to get everyone to like me, well I done that up until I started my new job and I couldn't stop it. I really did not like that about myself at all, why was I trying so hard? I wasn't in high school, I didn't need to be popular, fuck sake in high school I didn't even try to get people to like me so why was I doing it as an adult? It's totally mystifying but thankfully I don't do that now. I'd much rather people didn't like me for the person that I actually am rather than them like me for the person that I'm not. Now that I do understand because it's almost became like a mini-mantra that I practise, I think it's a good one as well because I'd rather be natural than to pretend to like someone or fake laugh at a joke that I just don't find funny. Seriously I'm thirty-three, I need to stop acting like I'm thirteen when it comes to new surroundings and new beginnings. So, that is definitely enough of the negatives, I know I said earlier that I didn't think I'm a good guy but I really am. I mean I am one of the good guys and that's one of the reasons I've got so many great people around me. I attract people to me and I think I just have something that is natural to me, now I know I said something different earlier but I have to have something, I don't have the kind of friends that I have if I'm an arsehole. I treat people how I like to be treated, I listen, I'm attentive and I'm a fucking good laugh on a night out. I also have a tremendous/inhuman amount of patience, I'm not even kidding I have tolerance and patience above human limits, I don't know how but I just do, it's just my luck I have 'superpowers' that would make me the worst superhero ever. I mean you have Superman, Batman and then you have me, 'Super Patience... Man', I bet I'd have one of those costumes where I'd have a cardboard plate with holes cut out so I could see, stupid cheap green tights and the classic white pants over them. I mean what would my purpose even be? (In heroic voice) I am Patience Man, I am here to rid the world of mis-understanding and... Oh fuck that, even I'm fucking bored of that and I've only just thought of it. So yea' I wouldn't be a great superhero but I do actually and genuinely have an inhuman amount of patience and tolerance, it serves me well. One of the main reasons that I've been able to build up my strength is because I've been focusing a lot more on my positives rather than my negatives. Although I don't have my own place just now I still find reasons to look forward. I need to look forward, now I don't like that word, 'need' but it's true, I do actually need to start looking forward, the time is right for me to start looking to the future, I have spent the majority of my life looking back and to be honest I'm absolutely fucking sick of it, has it got me anything? No. Has it been healthy for me? No. Has anyone ever achieved anything whilst constantly obsessing and focusing on the past? Absolutely fucking not. So why have I been so focused on it, what has me pointing a laser beam at my past and constantly bringing it up actually proven? It's proven absolutely fuck all. I don't want to be seventy and looking back thinking 'what if': - What if I just embraced life instead of worrying? - What if I accepted my past is my past and can't be changed? - What if I had lived a little I don't want to be that guy. I don't want to live a life with regret, fuck me I've got more regrets than I care to count. I don't need another thirty/forty years of them. Fuck that, I won't allow that to happen, I've been building my strength up over the last six months and the time is right for me to not only take control but to start living my life, I don't want to live in fear any more. I won't. Another problem I have is that I never know what I want and I never seem to settle in one place for long, when I'm in the house I want to go out, when I'm out I want to go home, when I'm in work I want to be outside, I just don't know what I want to be it. I'm constantly wishing time away and I don't like it. I think a lot to myself that I should be living in the now, living in the present because there's going to come a day when I don't have the luxury of time. Once again and it's a recurring theme throughout this but it's about mindset, I'm the one that controls my emotions, I'm the one responsible for managing myself daily so ultimately it's up to me. I know I'm making this sound super simple and I know it's not but you get the jist. I still really don't like myself, not as much as I should, I still think that I've got a lot I need to address before I would be content within myself, although I've made a lot of progress I wouldn't say I'm happy. I wouldn't say that I'm unhappy but I'm not content, I'm not satisfied, I still drive myself nuts sometimes with my thought processes, I still wander and lose control of my thoughts, I'm absolutely fucking terrible at concentrating, I can concentrate for so long and then I just switch off, I start daydreaming and wandering away to what I done at the weekend, what am I doing tonight, I look at people and I often ask myself what's going on in their head, what are they thinking, what's stressing them, what makes them tick. I spend a lot of time thinking and imagining what other people are going through, I can't stop it. When I'm on the train I like a lot of others participate in the sport of 'people-watching', I'm intrigued by people's individual mannerisms, from the way they sit down to the way they communicate with one another, it's just something that interests me, once again I don't know why. It's not easy to change engrained thought processes and it's certainly not easy when you're not happy within you. Is this an admission that I'm not 100% happy with myself at the moment? From what I've started writing in the previous paragraph I would have to say yes, yes it is. That right there is a fight I think I'm just always going to have, I'd love to sit here and say that I am completely happy and completely contented but the truth is, I'm not. When I was eighteen I started writing and when I say writing I mean poems and things, not writing as I am now. Over the space of ten years I had well over one thousand things written down and the majority seemed to focus on one thing, how unhappy I was. A lot of my writings hammered home the fact that I was deeply unhappy, at one point in 2007 I had actually written a sort of suicide note saying goodbye to everyone, the writings in that were very concise, honest and to the point. I guess if you're writing something like that you really have to be honest. Unfortunately I scrapped all of my writings after I nearly committed suicide in 2011, I felt that if I didn't have the writings then I wouldn't refer back to my past, the logic was there but I'm not sure it really made any difference. I'd love to say it did but here we are four years later and being honest I still have similar struggles to what I have them. I mean the stuff that I'd written wasn't clever, it was just basic rhyming so for example I'd write something like: 'These days they just get longer, my head just isn't changing I'm tired of putting on this front, this happiness I'm feigning I wish that I was better, I wish I wasn't such a stranger My strength is slowly waning, I think my life's in danger'. I mean it's not brilliant but it had a simple structure to it, it did also help because it forced me to think about what was actually going on inside of me. I don't know, do I really want to start digging this up again? I'm not sure I'm ready for it but then this links back to not knowing what I want, it's like The Clash with 'Should I Stay Or Should I Go', I don't fucking know and it really pisses me off, I don't think I should think this much, in many ways I'd love to just be an airhead, just having the wind whistle between my ears, not think of anything and just live a life. I mean really that sounds brilliant instead of my head, I hate the fact I can't switch off and I really mean that. When I said this was going to hurt right at the start I knew there was going to be a point where it was going to start really hurting, I'm at this point because what I'm basically saying is that I am not happy with myself, I kind of thought that I wasn't but this has confirmed it. I mean maybe this is what my life is going to be about. Maybe I'm just always going to be on the edge, stuck in the middle of happiness and struggle, maybe that's my place, maybe that's where I'm going to have to fight my battle from every day. Yea' actually this is really beginning to hurt, I feel like I'm pressing really hard with a salt covered finger into what I thought was a healed wound. It's not a healed wound, it's still open and it still feels raw, I wasn't prepared for this, I thought I was passed this, I guess I wasn't, I'm not ready and it may not be a bad thing, this brings me nicely onto my next major struggle... Alcohol... Oh god this is a bad one, I have a really tempestuous relationship with alcohol, it's been the cause of so much of my problems and it's something I've got to constantly fight against. I can abuse alcohol quite easily and it only happens over the course of a couple of days, see that's another weight on my mind and yet something else that needs managed. It's fucking hard work because I know once I get started on alcohol I don't stop. It starts with a couple of pints and within a couple of days it can spread to having six cans a night, not just a week, a night. I like to have a couple of pints on my own, I actually do. As much as I like going out with people and having a laugh I do have to constantly find the balance between being around people and being on my own. Yet another thing that I've got to find a balance on, as this goes on I really want you to see just how much I balance daily, no wonder I have 'not so good days', due to the strength I've got that enables me to keep them from turning into bad days, bad days are just... death, those are the days where I just want to run away from everyone and dive under my duvet. I want to shut the world out, turn my phone off and just ignore everyone. These are the days where I DO NOT AND I WILL NOT TOUCH ALCOHOL. If I touch alcohol then I'd be as well just doing it, I done it once and I will never ever do it again. It was four years ago and I still remember it. I remember walking around Glasgow bawling my eyes out, I still remember posting a last picture on Facebook, I remember the clothes that I was wearing and I still remember every single detail of that day. Alcohol and bad days are the absolute recipe for my own personal disaster. I will never ever do that again. But going back to alcohol, I've got an example of just how dangerous a relationship I have with it. I finished training on Friday (22/05/2015) and went out bevvying with my training group, they're a great bunch of guys and I'd been looking forward to it all week. I went out at about 13:30 and I left at approximately 19:30, I lifted the wrong laptop bag as well, fanny. Now I'd had a good day, I didn't have any sort of clouds over me and I was in a good place. For absolutely no reason at all I started crying whilst walking down Sauchiehall Street, now I don't know what caused this, all I know is there were similarities to THAT day in 2011, not quite to the same extent but the tears were real and I felt miserable. Now that was on a day where I felt great and I'd had a great day, things can change that fast in my head so it's absolutely critical that I keep a really close eye on things. As I said, things in my head can turn not at the drop of a hat but pretty fucking quickly. Thankfully my bestie was on hand to come pick me up and make sure I was ok. It just goes to show you even when you think that everything is ok you've got to be really careful. Actually I'll rephrase that because that's not right. It just goes to show when I think everything is ok I've got to be really careful. I don't think I was particularly drunk, I reached my limit and for once I decided to go instead of trying to blitz my way through it. I don't know what happened although I have a theory. I've just started this job, (I may have mentioned this) I've kept my cards pretty close to my chest and on Friday I was passing my book around, the one I wrote six months ago. Now my theory is this, even though I didn't look inside this book, even though I didn't read the contents did they embed in my head and as my alcohol consumption increased did the thoughts amplify subliminally? Did they somehow get past me when I was busy getting merry? It may not be definitive but it's definitely plausible. Something must have happened because I went from happy to crying in the space of a seven minute walk. The mind truly boggles, well.. mines does anyway. Maybe it would be better if I gave up alcohol? I mean looking at all I've been through it's been a constant throughout it. I don't know if it's been the actual root cause but it's played a significant part in my mental capitulations over the years. Maybe I just need to get a better handle on it, fuck off who am I kidding I depend on alcohol too much to give it up. I'm not even going to try to kid myself that I'll give it up because I just won't. I mean really Davy,

don't kid yourself or anyone else. You'll notice a key word there when I

was mentioning alcohol. I didn't say I 'enjoy alcohol' too much, I said 'I

depend on alcohol too much' and that is exactly what it is, it's a

dependency and one of the reasons I'm glad I don't have thousands of

disposable income is I would blow it on alcohol. (Remember what I said

when I left 3? Exactly) So I need to control my dependency because like

my happiness it's all about balance. Ugh I make my own head hurt at

times, I've just read the last two paragraphs back and it just confirms my

relationship with alcohol, it's fucked up. I don't know, maybe I should

actually look at it more and decide if I really want to pursue it. I mean, I

gave up sex pretty easily, surely alcohol should be an easier thing to give

up? Or am I looking at that in too much of a simple manner? I can never

decide if I'm looking at something too simply or too complex. Yet another

reason as to why my mind blows a fuse every now and then. I'm not sure I

want to continue on to be honest, since I've been writing I've noticed a

change in my mood, I can feel it, I don't know if it's because I'm actually

seeing what I've been thinking or if I'm digging deeper than I thought,

when I first started this I thought this was going to just be a

recap/building block of what I've done over the last six months, as it's turned out that's just not the case at all. This is getting deeper and I think it's going to get a lot more brutal, I can feel it. There's something deep down there, I can feel it's presence at the back of my mind. Oh well, better try and find it then eh? Point of reference, at the time of writing this it's 18:45 on 25/05/2015, I've just settled down with a couple of beers. I did say that I would inform you when alcohol was involved. It seems only fair that I keep my promise. So the last few days have been very strange. I wouldn't say I don't feel right, I'd say I feel ok, just not… right. Like I feel ok but I feel something, I can feel something that's burning away, almost like something faintly drilling at the back of my mind, trying to bore it's way to the front. Maybe this whole 'tearing myself down and rebuilding' me idea wasn't so good after all. I think a better way to word it because of the way I'm feeling is I am un-hinging myself and then trying to re-hinge myself, that's how I feel at this exact moment. I'm not going to lie I don't really feel anything at the minute, I just feel… I don't know what I feel, I'm having trouble really telling you how I feel, I'm trying to work it out but there's just nothing there. I mean I feel good about going back to work tomorrow, that's a start. I'm looking forward to seeing the guys, I've had three days off and they've been ok. I mean apart from crying on Friday night after leaving the pub yea' it's been a good one. I mean it has been ok, I think maybe I drank too much and was thinking about the book? I mean this was the first time I've been in public and discussed it since I wrote it. Also alcohol was involved so maybe that's what caused it? I'm still trying to decipher that one, I keep playing it over and over in my head and to be honest I'm still no further forward with it. The problem is that I can't leave it alone, I've got to just nit-pick it and analyse it, I've got to look for a point, I feel like a really bad version of Columbo, like a REALLY bad version. I'm no further forward so I'm going to try and leave it. I mean it's happened, it's in the past, I can't change it. I mean.... that's where it needs to stay. *takes a sip* I think I'm making things too complex again, I'm burning through mental resources un-necessarily and looking for things that really don't matter. I mean why am I trying to run over events with a fine tooth-comb when I don't really need to. All that I am really doing is using up energy that could be better saved for when I really need it like a not so good day or worst-case scenario a bad day. That's really been a theme of today, I've not really been thinking a lot but I feel tired mentally, I mean that may have something to do with the fact I'm writing all of this but I don't think it is. Even though I've literally just said I'm using up un-necessary energy and I need to save it I'm still using it. 'I'm still thinking and pondering, I'm sitting and wondering, I'm waiting and watching, for the thoughts that are walking Why won't this go and leave me alone, I want to stop thinking, and be on my own.' Ugh I'm getting annoyed with myself now. I hate my mind. No doubt it hates me too.

I fantasise a lot, I often come up with scenarios that are never ever going to play out in my head. I hate them but I can't stop seeing them. One that really pisses me off is when I wake up in the morning. I go through my morning routine, I get up, wash my face, shave my head and then have breakfast. Then for no plausible reason I fantasise about taking a penalty kick and doing a backflip in front of a cheering crowd. I mean... What the fuck? What is that? That makes no fucking sense whatsoever.. What am I even thinking, that's never going to happen. But most mornings it comes into my head, eventually I forget it and get on with my day. See stuff like that really screws with me because I'm not analysing everything but my brain comes up with this really stupid fantasy. I've got another one. When I listen to a particular group of songs I imagine it's me singing it on karaoke and I reduce people to tears, I MEAN WHHAATTTTT! Oh fuck off Davy what the fuck is that, that also makes no sense, the songs I do this to are: 'Umbrella' by 'Rihanna' 'Gone Away' by 'The Offspring' 'My Heart Is A Fist' by Papa Roach I don't play these songs now because I'm so tired of playing out that 'fantasy', see that's the type of shit that's going on inside my head, that's not normal, I can't convince myself it's normal. Do you know what I've started doing to try and block these stupid things out? I've started focusing on an imaginary pink ball at the front of my head, not only does it divert your focus away from stupid thoughts and fantasies but it also comes in handy for making yourself look blank. It comes in handy on the commute to work, I HATE business conversations at 7:47 in the morning. Seriously mate, shut the fuck up or I'll beat you to death with your own laptop. I need a huge mug of coffee before I can do anything in the morning. Listening to conversations about spreadsheets, projections and calendar appointments before I've had coffee is a very dangerous game to play. You are taking your life in your hands when you do that. Another thing that annoys me on the train is people that have full blown meetings over the phone before 8am.. Seriously mate/hen get a life. It can wait until you get into Glasgow, trust me it's not going to go away. I swear a lot of them are on the phone to their voicemail or something trying to look important, I have my doubts about people having these conversations THAT early in the morning. I think I'm just not a morning person, I'll rephrase that, I am fucking not a morning person, I generally come to around 12pm, that's when I start being productive, either that or after my third coffee. I've never really been one for small talk, I can be quite fidgety, I don't really have any confidence in my small talking skills at all unless I'm in the pub in which case I never fucking shut up. I do prefer myself on a night out, I'm a much more entertaining guy after I've had a few beers on a Friday! In general though I'm just not good at small talk, I try but I'm much more comfortable just sitting listening to people rather than getting involved. I always think whatever I've done is boring but then a lot of that links back into how I'm envious of other people. Nine times out of ten I have a perfectly valid weekend, I either go and practice snooker or I veg and play xBox, sometimes I meet my bestie and we hang out for a bit. Some weekends I'm actually quite productive and sit down and do budgets for the month ahead. Ok, that falls into the one out of ten category, I'm not going to try to kid anyone, that is boring as fuck. I don't know what it is but I just can't seem to maintain my confidence, I suck at eye contact as well, I always look away, I think it's to do with the fact that there can be such a thing as too much eye contact? Like someone totally staring through you, yea' I don't wanna be that guy, no-one wants to be that guy. So I've been doing a lot of thinking over the last couple of days and there's one thing I'm going to do on Thursday (Payday! Yey!) and that's buy a pair of big baggy trousers with chains on them, they make me really happy and I would say I've sort of lost my identity a bit without them, I dress nicely now but I don't want that all the time. I want to cut about with them on, have my music turned up and just be that little bit different. I know for a fact that's just not helped me confidence wise, I'm at my best when I look different, I definitely don't feel at my best when I 'look nice'. I mean it's ok, I always present myself nicely enough but I'm not like anyone else, I want that little bit of individuality again, it's a nice feeling to not feel like a clone of the person next to you. Actually the more I start thinking about this the more I want to think about piercings and tattoos. I'd love some new piercings and tattoos, that could be a plan but Thursday is a little bit of time away so I'll wait and see, definitely buying the baggy jeans though, those things are the fucking mutts nuts! Now that's interesting, just typing that I'm going to buy a pair of baggy jeans after payday has perked me up a little bit. I'm actually quite looking forward to that because they do actually make me happy. They're not for everyone I agree but each person has their own thing that makes them happy. For me it's definitely simple, baggy jeans, a t-shirt with a band slogan on it and a pint in one of my two favourite pubs in Glasgow, Rufus T Firefly or the Solid Rock Café, both pubs I frequent and I love them, mainly just because of the awesome tuneage that's played in both establishments. I've spent many a night there with friends. If you've never been I'd highly recommend them! I need to find some inspiration from somewhere, it gets pretty tiring constantly fighting with yourself, analysing everything you say and do. I need to try to find something that's going to serve me well in life, not something like a mantra but something that allows me to live instead of exist. That for me is a big thing. I don't want to hit sixty, seventy or eighty, looking back and realised that I didn't live my life, I existed it. That for me is not how I want to leave my legacy, I want to leave behind a lifetime of great memories and this is why personally my battle with depression is something I've chosen to write about. I've tried different ways of dealing with it in the past and none of them have worked if I'm being honest. I've tried therapy, I've tried talking to friends and I've even had professional help. I'm not saying it didn't help but I thought by this point I would feel better than what I do. Ugh that sounds like I'm being ungrateful, I don't mean it to sound like that, I'm grateful that so many people have invested so much of their time in me, I just can't shake that feeling that there's something inside of me that's different to everyone else. I think there's a lot I can give to people but I just need to unlock it, there's definitely something yearning inside me, something that says I can do more but quite what that is I don't know. God knows I'm trying to find it, I've spent fifteen years on an emotional rollercoaster and to be honest I think I'm going to be on it for the rest of my life. Maybe I'll never find it, maybe I'll search and search with no luck. Maybe I'll find something, something that I can hold onto and use for the rest of my life. I genuinely don't know, if I did then I wouldn't be sitting here clawing at my mind trying to get in. There's a point actually, remember what I said at the start about my levels of empathy? It's not just my empathy that's heightened, I feel so much compassion and emotion, I wish I could explain what I feel, I could try but I'd be here for one hundred years, I'll try to give you an insight into the emotion part, it happened two minutes ago so while it's fresh and here's how it broke down. So I was writing the paragraph above when my Dad came in and said he'd managed to find a recording of a TV show that he thought he'd deleted, so I went in, thanked him and watched the end of it. The end scene is magnificent, I don't know if I'm allowed to mention the name of the show so I won't. But the end scene and the accompanying end song that led to credits caused me to go into a stare, the music hit me really hard and I could fill every note, every word and every drumbeat fill my head, it washes over me like a wave, it moves me without trying, it fills my very soul with hope and it makes me forget what

I'm worrying about. That's how quickly it happens, certain songs played at just the right time can just make my heart sing, they can just alleviate me from my worries and take me to a place where nothing matters but as I say it's all about timing. I can listen to the one songs one hundred times but unless it's at the exact time that I need it then it's just a song, granted that song might be great but it doesn't give me that freedom, that release. Right now it does and I've not had that for a while. I feel moved, light, floating, I feel as nothing matters, these moments are as important to me as a good nights sleep, with moments like this I can hope again, I feel the freedom of the bars, the crescendo of the vocals, the loving caress of strings and I feel a heart soaring, I feel my heart soaring. I feel good, I feel strong and I write in time with the music. I share a very special bond with certain pieces of music and as of now I'm in time, I'm in tune and nothing can ruin this moment. Just to put into perspective this one moment has the potential to change the course of my next month or so, that's how important these bits of timing are in my life. I absolutely cherish these moments because they don't come around that often, I couldn't even put a number on it because it happens so little. All I know right now I have been carried skyward and I feel like flying. I feel my wings spread and everything lift. It's magical, spiritual and it's happened just when I needed it, when I was beginning to wane a little. I'm powerless when my mental strength starts to wane, the harder I fight, the worse it gets. I've got to let my not so good days just run because it's better for me. If I try and fight, I make my mental state worse, I know it's coming so I cocoon myself up and wait for it to pass. How could I describe it. It's like another layer appears between me and my mind, it locks me in and doesn't allow me to communicate freely. It walls me up and stops me from being. I've got sit inside my mind for two to three days, let it run and then I'm fine. Now I mentioned earlier about warning signs, I heed them, if any of the warning signs appear then I obey them, they advise me that trouble is coming and I'm glad they do because I get some time to prep, I get some time to ready myself for the coming days, my friends understand, my family understand, my work colleagues understood. This has yet to happen in my new job so when it does I'll have to be brave. It's actually quite a surreal place to be when the not so good days hit. My level of focus just skyrockets, although I can't physically engage in small talk my focus to my work increases ten-fold, it allows me to do what needs to be done but nothing else. I do not question my mind through this time, I'm indebted to it because it's warned me of an impending danger, to this extent me and my mind have an unspoken agreement. He has been so kind to warn me of some unpleasant times on the horizon, I do not speak ill of him and he processes what needs to be processed until I am well again. There are times where me and my mind do work together as a single entity, I like it when we do because we know what needs to be done, I'm thankful to him because he does me a favour, I should maybe be a little more appreciative of my mind. Maybe he'll take this as a thank you, I hope he does. That's the thing though sometimes there is no trigger, sometimes it just.. happens and then I'm left sidestepping and dodging anyone and everyone, sometimes there is just no reason for it. It just engulfs me and I have no choice but to deal with it. I've no choice to accept it and then run with it. These are the days when I'm glad to be on my own, everything makes sense in my head, because of the barrier goes up no thoughts get out, none come in and none cycle, my thoughts don't get into their speed cycle and so I can sleep for a few nights. It's almost like the not so good days are resting me, taking control for a few days and just slowing things down. I'm not going to lie, sometimes I do like these days, they give me time to myself and they give me time to re-energise and re-focus for when the thoughts start their cycle. That is by far the hardest thing I've got to control, the not so good days are more than manageable but when I can't get a single thought that's when I'm in danger, that's when I need someone around me because I'm stuck, I don't have that protection anymore, my mind has no firewall so the thoughts do as they please, they race out of control and they create a huge internal vortex, I can't settle, I can't focus and I can't sleep, god I fucking hate these days, 'the cycle' doesn't break and it just gets faster and faster, taking every positive thought I've had/I have and just sucking it into the vortex, swallowed whole and not to be seen again. This for me is hell, there is no set routine, there is no kill switch I can engage, whenever I close my eyes all I see are the thoughts, all I see is a hurricane enveloping everything and all. Every single thing I've done wrong in my life comes back at me, taunting and haunting me. Raping me and robbing me, I sit for hours just looking out a window, praying for this to stop, internally pleading with my mind to stop this from happening, our relationship has fractured, I've had no warning so this is all on me. My sleep is broken and deep, my eyes are heavy and bagged. I'm not resting and one day is running into the next without a break. I've had no time to recoup, it's straight into battle and slowly but surely my mental strength starts to suffer as a result. I have to focus so much of my strength on quietening the cycle that it leaves me little else for anything else. I've seen it effect my work, my personal life and before I took my vow of celibacy it even affected that as well. Granted that was a rarity but it still impacted. This for me is the part of my depression that I fear the most, I am so scared of it because I know it's the most susceptible state of mind that I can be in. That's normally when suicidal thoughts start to form and those take a tremendous amount of hard work and controlling. I could tell you just how hard I work at this but I don't think you would ever appreciate just how much effort I've got to put in to stop them. That's not a dig at you, if it comes across as that then god I apologise, I'm trying to convey just what happens at the height/depths of my depression, when I'm at my absolute worst and the tears won't stop flowing, the tears just keep coming and coming. They need to being honest, referring back to how much emotion I feel it's only natural that it erupts at some point, thankfully it happens when I'm in the cycle stage, if I feel it's going to help I'll watch Turner & Hooch, that film guarantees me tears so I put it on and let the tears flow. Am I ashamed to admit this? No. I need to do this because it does help, there is no kill switch, there is no way out. All I can do is sit, barricade myself in and pray that this alleviates, pray that this lifts. Depression is a horrific illness, I mean it just flat out sucks because it can strike at any given point, fortunately the majority of my episodes strike after some warning but when it's cyclic, I'm pretty much fighting it 24/7. Fuck that takes it's toll. In work it's a horrific discussion to have to have with a manager. I mean it's just not one I'm ever comfortable having. Physically I'm fine, I look ok but if I've got armageddon kicking off in my head then it's best for me to say what's going on. Now I've been fairly lucky in the fact that when it's struck me in work I've had the warning so it's been relatively low-key. I am dreading getting the cyclic depression at work, that would be an absolute horror situation and an absolute fucking nightmare. I'm still scared about opening up to people I'm not comfortable with about my battles, I think that's perfectly natural though, I wouldn't feel comfortable just walking up to someone and blabbering all of what I've written above, I have to manage each person individually. Some people get to see everything that happens and some people only get told at surface level 'I'm not feeling too good today', that's completely deliberate on my part because not everyone needs to know exactly what's happening inside of my head. There is one person that knows everything that goes on inside my head, just one person and my parents don't even know everything. I choose to keep some information from them because this is my battle. I have to fight this and as long as they know I'm either coping or having just one of those days then that's plenty. I would say if I was to describe my 'depressive personality' I'd definitely say I'm an 'introverted depressive', I like to keep everything to myself and unless I'm specifically asked for info. concerning it then I'll volunteer nothing. I think with the way my mind works it's best I keep things to myself, I delete my Facebook app for a couple of days, I delete any sort of messaging tools that I have and I just wall up until such time I'm ready to emerge again. I used to be the opposite where I shared everything with everyone, that didn't work because not everyone needs to know everything. I have a very close circle of friends that I would trust with anything, if they ask or I need to talk to them they get everything. As I say if I do need to have 'a conversation' with a manager within my new role it's going to be dependent on just what kind of depression I'm suffering from. Hopefully I never have to have the conversation and I can just.. work. That being said though I still think there's a negative stigma surrounding mental health and I don't think it's particularly anyone's fault. It's just.. hard saying to someone 'I don't feel good today' or 'I'm suffering today'. I find it hard, to this day I still find it hard to say to someone because the first thing they do is worry, it's perfectly natural because you're basically saying 'I'm not right' even though nine times out of ten it's temporary. I'll give you an example. Around the middle of December I made four videos and posted them on YouTube, they ranged from talking about depression to my own struggles with depression to the fact that I felt I was coming out of depression, I think one of them I made when I was drunk.. (cringe..) But I made those videos around the middle of December and less than two weeks later I had been hospitalised once for almost attempting suicide and then again for actually attempting suicide. So when people get worried I completely understand why they do, it must be terrifying for them to know a person is either contemplating or saying they're actually going to do it. I mean that's what I done and I worked my friends and family into a frenzy, I didn't mean to but as I said earlier, I'd had enough, my reasons for living no longer outweighed my reasons for dying, I had ran out of strength, I'd had too many cyclic days and I'd fell into the alcohol trap, my head was fucked and unfortunately I had decided that I'd had enough. I'm not proud of it but I did say that I didn't know if I was going to make it out the other side. I wasn't being dramatic, I was being factual, I didn't know where my battle was going to take me and unfortunately I did give in, I succumbed and I wanted out. I'm not ashamed though, I sit here with my head held high because that battle was personal to me, yea' ok I didn't beat it through sheer willpower but I did eventually beat it and start working towards recovery and re-habilitation. I think it's testament to the sheer amount of mental strength that not only did I beat it but nearly three months to the day that I'd attempted suicide I then applied for, prepped for and then managed to secure the great job that I'm in now. That's what gets me through not so good days, the sheer amount of strength that I have, I managed to come through a horrible period of my life and I didn't just come through it, I also managed to gain employment with a great company and get a great job in Glasgow. Just on the subject of things not helping me do you not what doesn't help me, when people don't tell me something directly. See if you need to tell me something? Tell me it. Honestly I'm thirty-three years old, I'm pretty sure I can handle it. I mean things like if someone doesn't like me or they have something to say to me. Just come out with it, I hate pussy-footing around, I'd rather just be told something than just sit there and wonder what's going on. Honestly, I'm not going to act like a thirteen year old who's been killed playing Call of Duty, I'm a big boy, I can take whatever is thrown at me, trust me. I've been dealing with this crap for fifteen years, I'm pretty sure I can take anything thrown at me, positive or negative. I just somehow feel as if I get babied, like given watered down versions of things. Trust me, if you've got something to say then please, do me a favour, just give it to me straight. Don't really know where that came from to be honest, just must have been one of those things that has been building up y'know? So hopefully you'll remember when I said under the right conditions beer allows me to open up just enough? I feel exactly what's been written was exactly what I wanted to get out, over three hours I had two beers and between that and the music from earlier it's allowed me just to cut myself open and bleed a little bit out. If someone who'd never suffered with depression was to come up and ask me 'What is depression like' I think I would struggle to answer, I mean I know what it's like but could I honestly get across to someone who's never struggled exactly what it's like? Could I encapsulate it? Could I describe it? Do you know something I'm not sure I could without making it sound dramatic. I wouldn't be trying to make it sound like that but I think it would come across as that. How would I describe it, well.. what if I was to say it was like walking into a really strong headwind or trying to push a car up a really steep hill? Would those examples work or would that be too simple an explanation. I mean is the definition of depression constant? No, it's not. I wonder should I maybe use the example I used above that's personal to me and the differences where I have 'warning sign depression' and 'cyclic depression'? Would that maybe be too much? Do you know something I don't actually know if I could describe it. I mean don't get me wrong, I'd give it a fucking good go, there'd be no doubts about that. I guess it would be dependent on the person, one thing I do know about depression is that lots of people suffer from it. I know I mentioned it in my last book but the death of Robin Williams really hit me hard. That's what started things off again, that one incident started the cycle again. I was going along ok, ok I was on a bit of a drinking spree but I was managing, then I woke up one morning and heard that Robin Williams had died. Now Robin Williams was in his sixties when he died, I think what that said to me was that I was never ever going to beat depression, I could never outrun it. Up until that point I had convinced myself that I had defeated it. Now when I say I'd defeated it I'm referring to the point in 2011 where I almost attempted suicide. I'd made great strides since then and I was doing well, yea' I still had 'off-days' and 'not so good days' but no real bad days to speak of. That one incident I can pinpoint as where my thinking patterns changed. I wasn't the same internally, I didn't think the same after that, I started to worry, I started to wonder if this was going to come back again. What would I do if it hit me in my fifties? Who would I have around me? Would I die alone? Would anyone actually care? What if I'm miserable for the rest of my life and I'm constantly trying to outrun the reaper? But... I've beaten depression haven't I? I mean I've came close to suicide but I've not done it, 2011 is past so surely I've nothing to worry about? WRONG. I started to worry. I started to worry a LOT. I started drinking more, I was having not so good days but ignoring the warning signs that my mind was mapping out for me. I wasn't sleeping. So looking back not only did I ignore my warning sign depression but I also chose to ignore the far more serious cyclic depression. I had started suppressing and that, well wow that worked out well didn't it. I started feeling unwell at the start of August, now when I state I was feeling unwell I am of course referring to my mental state, physically I was ok, just.. ok. The real danger sign came on 16/08/2014 of last year, I started writing poems down again, I wrote a few poems which pointed out quite clearly something wasn't right, once again though rather than facing the problem head-on I ran away from it. So in the months leading up to my breakdown on 01/09/2014 let's look at the timeline of just how things transpired: - Start to show signs of waning mental strength at the start of August - Robin Williams dies on 11/08/2014 - Symptoms of warning sign depression ignored - Signs of cyclic depression ignored - Writing about low mood and pain on 16/08/2014 - Drinking heavily from 16/08/2014 until 31/08/2014 So if you look at that you'll see it's a pretty fast decline. Now I'll be the first to admit I crashed through my warning signs and kept going, that was a mistake but that's just how quickly things can change, by the time 31/08/2014 came I was drinking so much that I wasn't even tasting the alcohol, I was drinking to forget, I had drank so much and suppressed so much that by the time I was waiting on the train to work on 01/09/2014 I was broken. I stood at the train station crying. I was thinking about suicide, I was thinking about jumping in front of the train, I was thinking how to say goodbye to everyone, my mind was shot and this was due to the culmination of events I've just described. I mean let's ignore events one, two, four and five and focus on the ones highlighted in bold, I CHOSE to ignore the warning signs, normally my friendly depression I decided to ignore my mind, it told me something wasn't right but instead of heeding, I ignored. Not only that…. Not only that but when I got my far worse friend Mr Cyclic I ignored that as well, to this day I will never understand what was going on in my mind to make me ignore both of these very clear depressive states of mind. I chose to plough on regardless and I basically fucked my mind. The increase in alcohol was massive as well so when you take all of those factors it's not surprising in the space of less than a month I was ruined. That timeline all links together, all of it added together was too much for me to take and by the time I got into work on 01/09 I was a wreck, I couldn't speak, I couldn't speak to my dear friend that sat beside me, god I couldn't even speak to The Samaritans to talk to someone about me wanting to commit suicide, it was that bad I just couldn't talk. My mind was shot and everything was fractured and broken. Everything was just burnt out, my wiring was gone, my links were all fried and by the time it came time to go home I just wanted to sleep. Now... I'm going to skip ahead here because the next two months were fine, I was well into a course of antidepressants, something that I'd been strongly against previously. I'd started to rest/recuperate and I started to feel a little better within myself, I didn't really see any of my friends that much though because my state of mind was still paper-thin and I was still highly sensitised to the world around me. Overall though I displayed good strength, I'd avoided alcohol and yea', I felt ok. I done the things that made me happy. I played xBox, I cleaned the house, I maintained the house and I ensured that everything kept ticking over. Now from 03/09/2014 I started seeing my GP weekly, I saw him every week without fail. Throughout this whole experience he is the one person that knows everything that happened, he got the whole timeline and every single rumble and tremor that I experienced. I'd like to thank him for his time and advice. He was an absolute rock and I will never forget all that he done for me. Things started going wrong for me when he said the words

'You can have a few drinks with these tablets', although it didn't happen instantly I began to crave alcohol more and more. I'd put in a lot of effort to ensure that I didn't touch alcohol as I didn't want it interfering with the tablets, I began with one can a week, then I was having a couple of cans a week, then I wasn't taking my tablets some days and then I was having two/three cans every couple of days. Yip unfortunately I was back on the booze and the recovery/recuperation had slowed. Although I never showed any symptoms of cyclic depression I was definitely having a lot of warning sign depression, I did heed it when it came and I pulled my alcohol consumption back but doing things in hindsight I would have definitely stayed off the alcohol. By the time I'd had my brush with suicide and my attempted suicide I was really drinking heavily again. I'm not proud of it and being really blunt in my criticism I was an absolute fucking idiot. You don't get any second chances, once your life is finished then that's it, it's game over, it's done and I never once thought of that. I couldn't think of that, I wasn't in the mindset to think like that. I…. I deeply and wholeheartedly apologise to everyone that was involved in my life at that time, it must have been an absolutely awful thing to have to deal with, although it wasn't much fun for me it must have been ten times worse for you. I'm sorry, I really am sorry. I AM SO SO SORRY, I HATE

MYSELF FOR EVER PUTTING YOU THROUGH ALL OF THAT. TWO NEAR

SUICIDES IN A WEEK EITHER SIDE OF CHRISTMAS. I AM SO.. SO SORRY. It's

true, I really am sorry for that time but what I'd ask people to bear in

mind is that I wasn't me, I was so far away from the person I am it wasn't

believable. I felt miserable, I felt vacant, I didn't feel stimulated, I just felt

tired, I felt useless, worthless, draining, not worth it, reclusive, distant. I

felt as if the world was better off without me, I was better off without me.

My family and friends were better off without me. I was a drain on all

resources, I wanted the world to empathise with me, I wanted the world

with me. I wanted... I wanted people to understand just what hell I was

going through. For the first time I was thinking of myself, for the first time

I was thinking just about myself. I was thinking about my needs, I was

thinking about trying to pull through this but I was failing, my recovery

had stopped, my respite had gone, I had used all of my strength and I had

ran out. I had exhausted all avenues, I'd used all resources and for the first

time, I allowed myself thoughts about dying, I'd softened myself up with

six beers and I had decided on 20/12/2014 I was going to be no more, I

said goodbye to my friends on Facebook and pulled out a small table from

the cupboard. I stood on it. I put one foot on the balcony. I looked down I

looked up, I looked down I went to step and then jump, this was it. At that exact moment the door went with a mighty thud, I stopped. I took myself down and I answered the door. I went with the paramedics and the police and I spent the night in hospital. I felt guilty, I felt sick and I felt horrid that I'd put my friends and family through that. My friends had called the emergency services as they'd got my address details through Facebook. Less than a week later it happened again only this time I took twenty-one anti-depressants at once, I'd overdosed and text my brother to say goodbye, he phoned an ambulance, I was back in hospital yet again, passing out and vomiting from all the tablets that I'd taken. I spent the night in hospital with my Mum by my side, I kept passing out so I didn't really say much, I was a mess, I just didn't know what to say, what could I say? I'd just attempted suicide. I had given up, I had accepted in my head that I was going to die. The point I'm trying to make is this. Depression is very much a state of mind, now quite what that state of mind is I can't answer conclusively. I can only speak from experience and my experience is that I get hit in stages. I get some severe and not so severe episodes. It's been five months since all of that happened and things are so much better. I'm staying with my parents until I can get on my feet in my new job and then I'm going to make the move to Glasgow, it's my favourite city and I love the nightlife. I know I'll need to be careful though because there are many pitfalls that I'll need to be wary of, mainly alcohol. I mean I will really need to avoid excessive consumption of alcohol. Things change so quickly in life and in my life I need to do all that I can to ensure I live a full and fulfilling life.

July 2015

It's like I'm trying to find perfection, it's an ache that never goes away and it's a complete, total mind cluster. I mean it never stops. Every day it's like I don't know how my head is going to react, I don't know what's going to happen and I'm going to try to be someone different to accommodate . I'm so scared to be myself it's galling. Why am I trying to be someone for everyone? Why am I trying to be twenty different versions of myself? Why can't I just.. be myself? I mean surely that's how it should be right? I mean it's not a radical concept, it's not new, it's not ground-breaking it's just how I should be. This isn't hard, I'm making this hard. I've been writing again, I bought myself a little book a couple of months back so I could document how I felt day to day, it started off well and within three days my mind went to shit. As always it started in a pub, shock horror of all shock horrors. It started off with me reviewing my previous workings, reviewing and thinking.. Then thinking and thinking, then thinking and over-thinking, couple all of that with alcohol and you have a perfect storm. I don't mean to be the person I am and I mean that, I know I have a lot going for me, it's why I have lots of people around me, lots of good people but the wiring inside my head seems to be getting more and more tangled but I'll come back to this later. I've decided writing this there will be no chapters, I don't want to be organised in my writing of this because quite frankly I want to speak from the heart here. I'm not saying the last two weren't written from the heart but after reading them and re-reading them I just don't feel they've captured what I want to say. Don't get me wrong I read them back and yea' they say a lot and I'm glad they're written but I'm missing something, there's something that's just not out, something that still eats away at me, something that slowly corrodes any happiness I build up and that is what I'm searching for. Whoever or whatever you are come out.. please come out.. So less than a week after finishing my second work I started writing again, I thought that if I kept my writing up I could better control all that goes on inside my head, in a way I think it did but the bad days I had at the start of June were really bad, I mean REALLY, REALLY BAD. Words/phrases like 'dysphoria', 'disaccociation', 'psychogenic amnesia' and 'de-personalisation' were present, I had shut down again and once again I was beginning to enter the abyss of depression and whenever that occurs it's inevitable that thoughts of suicide start to stir again. I feel I've gotten to a point with this that these types of thoughts are normal. I mean in my head they are normal because they're there that often it's just something I manage. In fairness I have been managing them well, I always find it easier to focus on my negatives as opposed to my positives though. I've always been the same, I've tried to change it but it's a hard habit to shift. I'll be upfront though and I will say I know it doesn't help me, focusing on negatives is never going to lead to a clean, healthy mind. Am I over-thinking again? Is this something that I should be seeking professional help over? Well, yea' the answer to question two is definitely a yes, question one I'm still contemplating over. I'll come right out with this right at the start so there are no misconceptions, I'm an alcoholic and it's something I will publically admit that I'm fighting, I've been hitting the bottle hard and that is something I've found hard to beat, I've found it hard being sober outside of work, drinking is what I do, it's how I've 'coped'/'dealt/ with the inner workings of my head, yip I know, it's not the way to deal with it but I have no real other interests to speak of. I just don't get why my life is so hard, there's no reason for it to be as hard as this, I mean there just isn't, I have a great setup but it's my head, it's what goes on between the ears that's causing my life to be all convoluted and distorted, it's not having that simplicity, that peace of mind, that little bit of peace inside to just enjoy things, I mean it's something I'm craving, I'd quite like to sleep more than what I do, I'd like to worry less than what I do and most importantly I would definitely like to drink less than I do. It's only because I've ran out of money this month (July 2015) that I've stopped drinking, pathetic eh? The thing is though is I'm at my happiest when I'm on my own drinking, reading that I think it's going to look like a contradiction but it's really not. It's the one thing I like doing because it allows me to tap into what I believe is my right mind and start dissecting all that's happening, there is a fine line I'll admit but it allows me to write and write and write, it can't be right... can it? It's hard though, I mean it's hard getting up in the morning when I'm having one of 'those days', the thing is they can come out of nowhere, it's like being side-slammed in a car and still having to go about my day as if everything's fine, that's the hardest part, that is by far the hardest part. I really don't want to have to fight this until I die but the thing is I think I'm going to have to. A thing that doesn't help me and it's entirely my own fault is I'm getting to the stage where I dreaded getting to. I've always said I didn't see myself getting past thirty-five I'm now thirty-three (and a half) and that age is looming, it's on the horizon and I hope that I not only see it but I live long after it. See stuff like that just isn't right but it's the way I think, I think at a very deep level and the way I see things confirms that to me. I don't look at things black and white, I see no grey areas I just see things as they are. Reading that back that sounds arrogant, it's not supposed to be it's simply meant to be a descriptive way of me trying to let you in. I need to let you in because if you see what I see then maybe you can see what I have to see, you see? To be honest I don't know if I'll ever be able to do this, I don't know even if anyone cares, I mean I'm just me, I am one insignificant person out of around seven billion, who cares really? I mean does anyone? I know I do and that's another part of my problem, I care WAY too much for everything. I don't have an off switch, I don't have the ability to zone out, I'm always on and I inevitably burn out from time to time, it's ok. I accept it. That's not to say it's all bad, I'm not trying to paint on a dark, depressive canvas, if that's the impression you get then I apologise, I'm not. I'm trying to paint a picture, an insightful picture. I'm not good that way, I don't really have the confidence to be myself, I live in my own bubble way too much, I hate it but when I come out of it, I just don't feel right. If I keep searching will I find an answer? If I keep digging will I find a breakthrough. If I keep writing will I uncover a truth and if I keep questioning and I do find what

I'm looking for will I like what I find? Ultimately what am I trying to achieve, am I writing just to vomit out all I suppress, am I trying to reach people? What am I trying to do? Can I be honest? I actually don't know, what I do know is that I'm trying to turn my mind inside out so I can have some peace, I deserve that much at least. I mean, there are times where I literally cannot function, there are times where I'm sat at the edge of my bed, looking out the window and I feel as if I'm actually trapped, I feel trapped both inside my head and inside my surroundings. I sit for hours and do nothing but stare, my head is too weighed down to do anything else. I put music on and I just sit. I don't reply to texts, I come off social media and I just.. sit, it's strange though because although I'm not allowed (by my mind) to do anything it's actually really calm inside my head, things make sense and I 'm allowed to breathe, I sit and stare but nothing happens inside my head. It's actually quite nice because it gives me a rare break from vortexing thoughts, worries and over-thinking. The hardest thing about is being around people when it happens though, I can't speak to them, I have no choice in it, I just have to sit and focus on whatever task I'm doing, I'm limited to oneword answers and just endless focus and concentration, I find it hard to look in one place walking. I put music on and I find myself gazing skywards, looking at clouds, I find myself looking from side-to-side and then down, then back up again, I'm lost in the music, it's almost like the music is coursing through my veins, I walk in complete rhythm to the song I'm listening to, my thoughts align with the rhythm and my head movements align with the pace of my walking AND the rhythm. It's actually quite surreal, I could walk for hours, I could write for hours and I can be at peace for hours. I can disappear, I can lose myself inside myself for days and just not care about anything else, I go back to sitting on my bed and looking outside the window again, it is actually a sweet place for me to be but I know I can't stay there too long, if I do I'll just never come back from it. I need to come back from it.. (wake up Dave, time to return) I'm terribly insecure in my appearance and my body, I never have liked how I've looked, it's just my way, I don't like myself that much, I'm pretty sure there's a link between that and my mental states, I just can't link them together. In fairness I am getting better at liking myself, it's something that's going to take a lot of work but I genuinely believe I work better being different from everyone else, I'm not good as 'another face in the crowd', I do like to be different and I'm in the middle of being that, it's a work in progress and as of today (12/07/2015) it's coming on fine, I just need to keep working on it, I'd like to point out I'm talking appearance wise, mentally I would love nothing better to be 'another face in the crowd' but at the moment I've got my appearance and my mental states the wrong way round. If I get the appearance bit right then I think the mental state will start moving in the right direction. That's the theory anyways, in practice I doubt it'll be that simple. I can dream though eh? I'm actually really impressed with myself, two-thousand words and not one single swear word, considering just how much I swear that is a feat. I make Gordon Ramsay look polite when I get going, can I write this and not swear once? Tall order but I'll give it a go. One of the many problems I have is my sheer inability to understand/perceive people. I can never just be one of the gang and just have a laugh, even when I do my head manages to mess things up, I actually think it's better for me to be on my own because then it's me and my mind, we can work our differences out and then if we can't then the only person it affects is me. I can write, I can lie down, I can have a bath, I can go for a walk, I can deal with it on my own and there are no casualties, people then don't have to worry about me, I HATE people worrying about me and I'll explain why: I appreciate the fact people care about me, I really do but I don't think it's fair on the people I love. I also don't like getting compliments, I really don't because I don't react well to them, once again I don't know why that's the case all I know is that it happens and I need to just deal with it. I find it tremendously hard to talk to people naturally, I always find myself struggling for words that sound right, I find myself grabbing sentences just so I can stay in a conversation and I don't like it, actually scrap that, I hate it. I strongly dislike the fact that I have to deal with this, I strongly dislike the fact that this takes over me and I just wish it would end. I don't wish my life would end but I wish this never ending tirade of mental abuse and violation would end, I honestly and genuinely think sometimes about running away, I think about where I could go to escape this but I know I never will. Maybe if I get my passport sorted, save up some money and then fly away I'll leave my mental capitulations behind, maybe if I start a new life then whatever mental problems I have to deal with will magically dissipate and I'll be happy, then I have to stop myself from thinking that way because I know that'll never happen and the longer I think of it the worse it's going to be when I'm dragged back to reality. See a lot of people dream for financial security, a lot of people yearn for 'the one', people dream of all sorts of things and you have to have a dream, if you don't have a dream then you're doing life wrong, everyone needs something to aspire to, something to achieve, to work for, strive for. My dream is to live in a mind that has minimal clutter, a mind that doesn't pollute the simplest thought, the simplest gesture, a mind that takes the good and shreds it into a million tiny pieces. I dream of living in a mind that is not only strong and robust but also allows for mistakes, a mind that allows things to happen naturally without setting off alarms, I YEARN for a mind that is free of breaking me down, wearing me down and shutting me down. I dream of having a mind that allows me to just simply be me and this is why I keep fighting, maybe one day I'll get my dream. I need to keep fighting, I WILL... keep fighting. Oh by the way on a side note the celibacy didn't last, I ended up having sex, oops. My intentions were good, just unfortunately my mind wasn't. Do I need a change of scenery? Do I need to change myself? Actually do I need to change anything? I tried therapy before but I got scared and ran off. Maybe I need to try harder, I've already came so far so is it mind over matter? Mind over mind? Mind over MY mind? How can I make my two frames of mind one, I've had it before but can I have it again? I'm pretty sure it's achievable, it has to be, I mean it's not impossible, it can't be. There's no way I can spend the rest of my life focused on my mind, I mean if I do that then I won't be living, I'll be managing thoughts and that's not living. I... I don't want to exist, I want to live, I'm thirty-three, (and a half) there's got to be something for me, has anyone seen the switch? You know the switch, the off switch, it's around here somewhere, I need to find it so I can enjoy life. It can't be healthy living like this, actually scrap that, it's not healthy living like this. It breaks my heart, I mean it honestly, one hundred percent breaks my heart to have to constantly fight something that exists only in my mind. I've hit the bottom, I've tried to commit suicide and it failed, I've hit the bottom so now I should be swimming for the top, swimming for the top of the water, I should be looking upward but yet I continue to waste my gaze looking sideways. Is this my life? Is it the mental rollercoaster, am I always going to be eternally looking up then down, I really hope not. I really hope that I live my life, I mean the desire is there, the hunger is there and the burning is there. There is fire in my heart, blood pumping through my veins, light in my eyes and desire coursing through every artery within me, like all things with me though I know this is temporary, I know this will disappear and I know at some point the darkness will be back, it's always there, just out of sight and blocking the light at the end of the tunnel. I've grown to hate it, manage it and hate it. I need an identity, I need to formulate a plan that allows me to keep my head in check, at the moment I feel as if I've got it on a leash that's a rotting rope, I don't feel I have any control over my mind and that's just not healthy for me. The thing is though I've tried not thinking, I've tried free-wheeling and just not putting any thought into my head and it just doesn't work, if anything I feel worse for doing that. I mean is any of this making sense? I'm not sure it is, oh well best keep going. It's like a weight, a weight that drags my eyesight down so I can't face myself in a mirror, a weight that causes me to constantly look down, to not be able to make eye contact with those I love. It's a weight that takes any happiness I have and anchors it so I can't reach it. In fact it's not 'like a weight', it is a weight, it pushes my head to my shoulders and makes day-to-day tasks an achievement should I achieve any. I remember I once went over forty days when I was at the height/depths of my depression, that's the hold this weight has over me. It makes even the most mundane, easiest tasks a chore, I have to reach deep down inside to have a bath, brush my teeth, cut my nails. I mean it has a hold on me, it has a vicious hold on me this and I wish it would just leave, I have no patience for it, I have no reason for it and I'm darn sure I have no desire for it. I'm at a point in my life where I feel like I'm a lot happier, I feel a lot more comfortable in my own skin and although I'm not one hundred percent I know it's getting there, I know I'm getting there and I see a lot more light than I used to. All in all I believe I'm coming out the other side, I keep pushing and fighting for it. It's a scrap but as someone that's used to fighting for things it's ok, I'm accustomed to it. I'm used to it and I'm going to give this everything I have, it just strikes out of nowhere though, the weight just clamps my legs like cement galoshes and just drags me under, leaving me at the bottom again and dreaming of swimming upwards again. It happens so quick, it cold-cocks me, it nullifies me, it takes anything good and turns it into a wretched, dehabilitating, numbing wreck of swirling thoughts. It somehow manages to find buried memories from my past, memories that I've fought so hard to deal with and it exhumes them. Infact it not only exhumes them but it resurrects them and places them right at the front of my mind again, when that happens I need to go into my cocoon, I need to ride it out and then I need to start the fight all over again. Starting from the bottom of the ocean takes a lot of preparation. Once 'the weight' lifts from me I can then start my fight again, I see it go, I see it float away, I know I'll see it again, I know I'll have to fight it again but for now it's released me so I can chip away at the galoshes and then start swimming again, there is no pattern to this, believe me I've tried watching it, I've tried it, monitoring it, looking at weather, diet, alcohol consumption and there is no pattern. Sometimes it just strikes, sometimes it hits, hurts and punches. Sometimes it beats me, sometimes it violates me and it ALWAYS floors me. It's like the flu only you can't see it. I see it, I see it from the bottom. I see my friends and family above, I see them above the surface, I see them

clearly, I reach for them and I know I'm miles away, I know I'm not going

to reach them, I know I shouldn't try to but I need to. I'm trapped again,

I'm under again, sometimes they're just out of reach and other times I just

can't see them. Even when I sleep I suffer, I don't rest, I never rest and I

get up the next again day, I get ready to face the day even though I'm not

ready. It's at times like this I think about running/swimming away. Maybe

the change of scenery……. Yea' I know, it's never going to happen, I've

accepted it and I've just got to accept it and await 'the weight'. It's funny,

the worst part isn't when it hits the worst part is knowing it's going to, it's

those two or three days of the thoughts mutating and taking on their evil

forms, it's the feeling that the swirling has started and bit by bit the light

is going to disappear, it's the preparations of the galoshes, the edging

closer to the cliff, the look down at the water and the recognition of the

spot where I'm going to be again. It's the realisation that soon enough I'm

going to be searching for my friends again, I'm going to have to cocoon,

I'm going to see nothing but black. It's the feeling of being trapped that

disgusts me, I can take being quiet, as I eluded to earlier I actually quite

like it, it's peaceful and actually provides me with some serenity, it

doesn't always. Sometimes it double bluffs me and my serenity and peace are eaten away by the vortex, sometimes it leaves me nothing. It's a hurricane and destroys anything and everything positive in my path. The water I'm trapped in is so cold, my head is so heavy, people are talking but I can't hear anything, people are laughing and I can't hear anything, people are around me but I'm not seeing them. All I see are the two blocks at my feet holding me at the bottom of the ocean, I'm waiting on the weight again, I'm just waiting for it to come below the water and leave me there again, leaving me to fight again. I've lost count of the times I'm left alone at the bottom wondering if I'm ever going to win, I've lost count of the times I've craned my neck skywards crying at the thought of having to deal with this. I've lost count of the amount of times I have felt susceptible, vulnerable, the times I've felt exposed, open, bared and unprotected to this. I have well and truly lost count of the amount of times that this has violated me and caused me to take on a whole different form, the amount of times I've lashed out at friends, I know it's not me but it disguises itself as me, guys it's not me, I'm trapped, lost in ocean of my own thoughts, please you need to understand this person that's snapping and faltering is not me, IT'S NOT ME. Guys help, can you hear me? I'm trapped, I'm lost, I'm drowning here, look it's me. I'm here you can't hear me though can you? I'm trapped watching this, I'm a spectator to my own destruction, I'm powerless and helpless. On top of everything else I've now got to watch myself implode, I hate it so much, it takes up so much of my time and takes up all of my resources, I am stretched to breaking point and does he care? Does it care? Of course it doesn't because it's doing the one thing it's always taken great pleasure in doing. It's destroying my happiness, it's destroying everything I've built up from the last time it hit. It enjoys ruining me and it loves the fact I'm watching whilst it…. no… HE loves it, he laughs whilst I'm stuck there, sitting on the ocean floor, he sits above me and pushes me down, he makes sure I'm grounded, glued, fastened, stuck, welded to the floor. I sit with my arms crossed staring at the ripples that flow around me, the water is getting cold again, he 's been here too long, he's been here way too long, why does he want me to suffer? What does he get out of it? Why is my happiness his enemy? What have I done to him, what did I do? Did I hurt you? Did I embarrass you? Please tell me, talk to me and tell me what I've done, you're absolutely and completely destroying any iota of happiness I have, that's all I want so why do you take it away. I hate you, I hate you so much but why do I even tell him because all that does is give him more enjoyment over me. He leaves me shipwrecked, he leaves me a broken mess and when he does finally leave me to break out I've then got to start all over again. I don't see him for days, weeks, months, sometimes even years but the longer he leaves me the more devastating it is when he appears again. Sometimes I stave him off, sometimes I pre-empt him, I feel the presence, I feel the heaviness of my feet, I feel a shiver, I feel something, I feel him, he's there, he's watching, he's always watching me and I know I've got to be ready for him to strike, he's dragged me under so many times that I know when he's about now. I've got to be most aware when I'm at my happiest, that's when he picks his time to strike. I know it is, he knows me intimately, he feeds of my misery so why strike when I've nothing to lose. He knows the time to strike is when I'm at my best, he ignores the cyclic, he ignores my bad days because I'm suffering, he loves watching me suffer, writing anything and everything to try and escape, he loves the thought of me wanting alcohol, he loves the thought of me thinking of suicide, he absolutely loves it and he loves watching me fight. What truly makes him happy though is him taking everything away from me. He loves when I'm at my happiest and then that's when he strikes, he contorts, distorts and punctures me, he stabs me right in the head and leaves me to bleed out, he leaves me with nothing, HE... LEAVES...ME....WITH....NOTHING, HE LEAVES ME WITH NOTHING, HE LEAVES ME WITH ABSOLUTELY NOTHING. How many times have I been left to die at his hands? Too many to mention. The fact that nobody really knows this I think shows good management on my part, either that or I'm a really good liar, actually I know that's not the case I'm a terrible liar. He is there though. I know he is and I know he watches me. He's like ... what is he like.. He watches everything I do and he bides his time, he is the hunter and I am the prey. I've fought this long enough so when he strikes I know what to do when I'm at the bottom again. I'm going to leave him for now, just thinking about him makes me shiver, he's creepy. So earlier I touched on writing just after I finished my second work, looking back at it it's scary how quick my thoughts changed, in the space of three days I'd went from writing things like 'Felt Good', this was on 30/05/2015 and within three days I was mapping these: - Dysphoria - Emotional Detachment - Psychogenic Amesia - Depersonalisation - Introversion - Splitting This was three days worth of writing where I didn't speak to anyone, I had to be locked away within myself trying to get to the bottom of what was happening to me. This is why I always need to be aware, I mean things took a turn over what turned out to be about four days, I look back at the writings and I can actually see when things started changing, it's a little un-nerving but at the same time I know that I'm likely to see that whilst writing . I know when I write that more often than not something isn't right, I'm not going to be as arrogant to say it's like a sixth-sense it's just a feeling I get. Bear in mind between the ages of eighteen to twenty-nine I had filled about ten notebooks with writing, I mean that's all I done and I could count on one hand how many writings were happy. They weren't and a lot of them were very very scary. At one point I'd written a suicide note and this was in 2006. So even when I was twenty-four the demons were there, infact looking back I'm glad I did write, after 2011 when I nearly committed suicide I decided to get rid of them, I don't know if I done the right thing, I think I did but I don't know. Might have been nice to check in with them and see if what I was feeling was similar to what I feel now. I wonder if 'he' has always been there, was it him that started messing me up at eighteen, was it him that started me wanting to be alone? Hmmm, I wonder, the older I'm getting though the more he is interfering , the more he is taking control, the longer this goes the harder I need to fight to keep him out, I need to keep him out because one day he's going to get control of me and cause me and my loved ones a tremendous amount of pain. I'm fighting hard, I'm fighting super hard to manage my mind, I'm fighting to control my alcoholism, actually writing this I'm also fighting the urge to swear, still haven't though, this could actually be the longest I've gone without swearing. There's something strange about trying to delve into your psyche, it's weird trying to tip it out for everyone to see, it's slightly off-putting but then I know in order for me to try and defeat/stave off this I know I'm going to have to. I know that it means I'm going to have to dig and already I know something I'm going to say that isn't going to be easy to read for me… I need to be on my own, I need to stay off of social media and I need to socialise with people when I know that HE isn't around, he caught me out a few months back and I won't allow him to do it again, I can't allow him to catch me out. I need to do things on my own terms but whether I do that or not is anyone's guess, I think it'll be highly unlikely because I know myself that I don't follow-up on things, I don't learn, I'm not half the person I think I am because I keep falling into the same traps, I'll go out when I'm not feeling well, I'll have too much to drink and I'll end up blowing up. I'm not learning and that's stupidity, it's first-class idiocy and it irritates me. I'm not stupid, I'm way better than this and ultimately I need to start heeding the signs, it's ok me writing and saying this but I need to start doing it, I need to start taking my own advice, it's ok when I'm giving advice but when it comes to me actually taking any I don't. That's bad, I can't afford to do that with all that goes on inside my head, if I'm ever going to beat this then I need to start heeding both advice and the danger signs. So today (12/07/2015) I've taken myself off of social media, pretty sure I've done this before and failed but as I'm writing this I'm actually saying this to myself I NEED TO FOLLOW-THROUGH WITH THIS', me and social media do not get on, I NEED to take myself away from it and I need to focus on myself, the world doesn't need to know everything I do and I certainly don't need to know everything it does. I'd be quite happy not knowing what people are doing so if I take myself away from that it should help. The thing for me is can I stay off of it? I'll need to, it drives me nuts and I probably drive it nuts. I need an identity, I need something to hold on to, I need to start work on being myself because at the moment I'm not. At the moment I alter my persona to fit in with people when I know I shouldn't, when I'm myself and this is in a working sense I'm very much tuned to my job, I find it easy to just get in and get stuff done, it's how I do things but I've found myself just inputting into conversations just for the sake of doing so. It's not right and I don't like it, I am so scared to be myself it actually sickens me a bit. There is nothing wrong with me being myself, I just get so scared to be it though incase people start thinking something's wrong and that's what messes me up. That sentence right there is a nail right on the head. I'm scared to be quiet (I'm naturally quiet) incase people think that something is wrong, that whole ethos is wrong, it's a crap theorem, it's a stupid equation, it's a totally crap way of looking at things, I'm better than that, that's why I need to start finding this clarity and peace of mind. If I don't I'm just going to think myself to an early grave and one thing I know for definite is this... He has absolutely nothing to do with this, this whole charade has been my own creation. I think it started when I left school and I started work, in high school I done ok, I was neither popular nor bullied, I just got on with things. When I started work I wanted people to like me so I sort of faked my personality, so I'd go on nights out and pretend I was this total rock and roller who liked nothing better than boozing and shagging, don't get me wrong, I do like these but they're not all I am. I wanted to be popular, I wanted people to think when they looked at me, 'legend'. In hindsight I'd play it entirely different because after fifteen years of not being me it's began to fester away at me, it's began to eat away at me and now I'm going to find it hard to change. Then again a question I actually need to ask myself is this... Who am I? As in, who am I because I don't actually know. Don't get me wrong it's not through lack of trying or through lack of effort but I genuinely don't know the guy that's staring me back in the mirror. There are many reasons for that though, to an extent I've lost my way a bit, my judgement is clouded, I overthink things to death and I've allowed alcohol to control me, gone are the days where I enjoy the odd drink, I now drink whenever I can, that's sad and it makes me sad actually admitting that I'm an alcoholic, there are no two ways about it, I am and it's something I need to address, it's something that I have started addressing though but it's something I need to stay on top of. I need to stay on top of it because when I come 'off the wagon' I come off of it hard. I get bored easy, I'm currently back staying at the folks and I drink out of sheer boredom, god knows what's going to happen when I get my own place, I really need to build up my mental strength for when that happens, I know what I'm like and I know by a long way that alcohol is my biggest vice. It's not my only one though, the fact that I don't really know who I am is up there, I have no identity, I have nothing else to differentiate me from anyone, it's almost like I'm a zombie, I just seem to exist with no real purpose, one day merges into another, it's then a week, then a month and before I know it I'm another year older and it's yet another year where I've not done anything of note. It kills me, it really does, I mean I genuinely feel as if I'm wasting my life.. I mean am I? Am I wasting my life? It feels as if I am but then I think of all that I have to contend with, I've said it myself I don't feel as if I'm connected the way others are so am I wasting my life or am I fighting for my life? I should really know the answer to this but I don't, I don't have the answer, I don't have it. I mean.... why don't I have the answer? I don't even know what I want, do I want a girlfriend? Do I want lots of money? Do I want a nice house? I don't know, again I.. DON'T... KNOW. It almost feels like there's a part of my mind that's locked, like it's been hidden away. The core is there but when it comes to me trying to work out what I actually want I can't tell you. It saddens me, it really saddens me that I can't tell you what I want out of life, at the moment, shortterm I'll take managing my thoughts and him. It's not exactly out of this world stuff though is it? I feel like I'm split into three different versions of me, the strong version, the weakened version and the reflective version. It's probably stating the obvious but the three parts never combine, each one makes up one third of me and at any one time only one part is in operation. Nine times out of ten it's either version one or version three that are in operation but when version two strikes it then the trouble starts. Although it's only one part of me the weakened version has various forms and versions and they range from under the weather to full on manic/depressive/suicidal forms, unfortunately when that version of me is operating it's hard for me to manage, I have to really grit my teeth and fasten my seatbelt because depending on the form I take even being around people takes a lot. It's a crippling state of mind to be in and I mean that. It manifests itself as different forms of depression and slowly but surely eats away at my strength. The only time I'm at the higher end of that scale is when 'he' appears, when he appears I know that I'm in trouble. This has been the first time I've been able to humanise him, probably because he's been on my mind a lot since I went off from work last year with depression. Mind you it was coming for a long time last year, I'd basically hid it for months and my drinking sky-rocketed, when that kind of stuff happens things just aren't right. I'd managed to blow a substantial amount of money over three months and to this day I can't really tell you what I actually spent it on, that didn't help but you know what really didn't help? Not talking to anyone, hiding it, burying it so everyone thought I was fine, I wasn't fine, I was the furthest thing from fine. I was in so much pain that I was suppressing the manic/depressive/suicidal forms of myself, to be honest I don't know how I lasted so long, it must have been about three months of carrying on the charade that I was ok, yea', that worked out well didn't it? I honestly wish you could see inside when I'm hit, see inside when I'm hurt. Physically there is no difference but mentally he caused me so much pain. Looking back I didn't realise just how much strength it took me to get through each day. Actually looking back I don't know how I managed to get through each day, there were a lot of days where I done nothing. I mean I done absolutely nothing. I spent my days either playing xBox all day and not moving or I spent the day wandering from room to room, I was almost in a catatonic state of mind, nothing was happening, I spent day after day sitting, I spent day after day looking out of my window, I spent day after day after day after day trying to figure out what this was. I spent so much time trapped in my mind that it changed the person that I was, I was trapped so much in my mind that I was not only at the bottom of the ocean when he hit me, by the end of December when I had my two suicidal episodes I was actually giving in to him. I had had enough of it. I spent over one hundred days chained inside my mind, I'd spent that long inside that I couldn't get out. By the time I had reached the middle of December I had no fight left, I'd fought and fought and I had nothing to give, it was by far the hardest thing I've ever done, by far the hardest decision I'd ever made but I'm glad I made it, it was the indicator I had reached the bottom and make no mistake. This wasn't a cry for attention, this wasn't me saying I needed help I want to make one thing painstakingly clear, that night I overdosed I fully intended on taking my own life. I had given in and I was tapping out, I had had enough, my mental strength by the end was paper thin, now for someone who prides themselves on their mental strength that is a hard thing for me to admit, I have no shame in admitting it though because after a lengthy battle I have to say I lost. By that time in mid-December I wasn't the same person, I wasn't the man that my family and friends knew, when I looked in the mirror I felt nothing, I had no care for myself, for weeks I knew I was running low on fight and the water was just below my chin, I felt the weight pulling and pulling and pulling and after fifteen years of wars I had eventually lost. The weights finally dragged me under and I began to slowly sank and drink my way to the bottom. I was drinking so much that I had lost the taste of beer, it was just a way for me to get away from my troubles, I was drinking so much in fact that it was routine for me to go to the shop and just buy six 660ml bottles of beer and just get drunk. I spent my final few weeks giving in and drinking my way to death, I'll admit it, I have to. I tried going online and pouring my heart out via online channels and making videos but it didn't help. By the end I wasn't even a shell of my former self, just a depressive alcoholic with nothing to take but pills. I took twenty-one pills all at once, I'd done it, I'd finally plucked up the courage to commit suicide, did it feel euphoric? No it didn't because after I'd done it I'd realised I'd given in, I'd succumbed, he had won and I could hear him laughing at me. I knew that by overdosing I had finally admitted he was stronger. I ended up in hospital vomiting as my brother had phoned an ambulance, twice in one week I'd ended up in hospital as only seven days previously I was one step away from jumping off of the balcony on my flat. Unless you suffer you can't possibly understand the sequence of events that take you there, that lead you there, the events and trauma and pain that slowly cut off every escape path and direct you to that. Unless you suffer then you'll never understand the thought of your very soul giving up and accepting that death is the only thing left. You'll never understand and if I can be one hundred per cent honest with you... .. I wish I couldn't understand it either. Depression is one of the most horrible things that you can ever encounter, it's one of the most debilitating, destructive diseases that you can ever suffer from. Depression is an evil, demonic disease that causes you to take different forms. It's an absolute horror, what really gets me about it is I know that I've been doing better, yes I've had not so good days and a few bad days but I know I'm never going to beat it. I now know the rest of my life I am going to have to always be alert, I'm always going to be watching for the danger signs. I know that through my thirties, forties, fifties and sixties I am going to have to be vigilant. I wish I was an airhead, I wish I had nothing between the ears, I wish that my spelling was bad, I wish that I had nothing going on so I could live a life of ignorance. I absolutely hate the fact that I have to manage three differing versions of me and I really hate the fact that I can't talk to anyone about it. I've tried, god knows I've tried to but I just can't open up. I've said it before and I'll continue to say it but I cannot talk to people about this because I feel as if it's not real, I don't believe people will be taking me seriously when I say what I've said above. I want to be completely open about this and the only way I can do that is to write, I think this is the way I'm going to have to deal with it, by writing. In many ways I don't think that's a bad thing, infact in many ways I think it's actually a good thing because when I'm writing I talk no- holds barred, I talk with no filter, no fear and I talk openly, honestly and freely. The hardest thing for me is always going to be managing it when I have to be around people, it's awful when I'm on my own in a social environment and I just cannot talk, it's gut wrenching knowing I'm going to have to sit for two to three days knowing I'm going to be on my own. I get home and it's not any better there, when this strikes I never want to be anywhere. When I'm at home I want to be at work, when I'm at work I want to be playing snooker, when I'm playing snooker I want to be at home and so on and so on. It is absolutely horrible, my appetite goes right down, my alcohol consumption goes right up, I don't take care of myself and I make the biggest mistake of all.. I block people out. How do I talk to people when I don't know what to say? How do I call someone or text someone and say 'I need to talk' when I'm scared to death of what's going to come out. When it comes round I think of suicide, it's part of my thought pattern when this comes around, I can't help it and it annoys me. When I broke down at work last year I tried calling The Samaritans but I just couldn't. I tried but when you're bawling your eyes out it's really not fair on the other end of the phone, they're just not going to be able to understand. I tried though, I mean I genuinely did try. A lot of the paragraphs I want to start with 'do you know what my problem is' because a lot of what messes with my head is to do with me, there is very little outside that interferes with me and I'll give you an example. Today is Sunday, Sunday the twelfth of July, I finished work on Friday the tenth of July and I was looking so forward to the weekend, now that I'm on the weekend I'm looking forward to going back to work and I am ninety nine. nine percent sure that as this week goes on I'll be looking forward to the weekend again, my point being this. I absolutely suck at staying in the present, I'm either wishing my time away whatever I'm doing or when he strikes I'm constantly regretting every single thing I've done in my past, I hate it, I absolutely frickin' hate it, it's something I've worked on but I just can't seem to do it. I'm also way too harsh on myself when it comes to making mistakes, I allow myself to get away with absolutely nothing, I make a mistake and I replay it and replay it and replay it, it's ridiculous. I over analyse myself on everything I do, I don't like the way I look and I never really feel right in my own skin. I know I can't change that one and as I said earlier I am working on that but it will take time. My point being this, I shouldn't be looking back and if I do I should be proud but I'm not, I have this empty/nothingness type feeling going on and it's almost like I've been numbed by anaesthetic, it's a feeling that just has nothing attached to it. It's dull, it's boring and I'm sitting here looking at this thinking how much further do I need to hate myself before I start appreciating me for who I am. There's a lot I can't change about myself, my hair isn't going to grow back so I need to keep shaving my head, I can't change my age because as we all know time is a constant and stops for no-one, I can't change what's happened in my past so there is absolutely no point in dwelling and revisiting/regretting. The thing that I need to look at changing is my mindset, or do I? Ninety percent of the time I have the right mindset, I'm positive, hard-working, friendly, organised and in control, it's just that ten percent when I lose control that I need to change. In fact even that's not true because in general even when I have bad days I still manage to control them pretty well. I'm confused, I'm genuinely and utterly bamboozled as I sit and write this. I don't even know if my mind is tangled or untangled, I can't tell you how I'm feeling because like I say I'm almost numbed. I've done nothing today, I've spent all day in my pj's playing xBox and I feel relaxed but something inside me is telling me I should have done more, should I have done more though? I mean, it's a Sunday so I should have went on a bike ride or went for a walk, instead I've drank my weight in coffee and basically tried to once again make sense of this chaos that rages within me. I wonder sometimes if I'm ever going to be able to make sense of it. I wonder actually if I want to make sense of it. There has to be something to it, I mean... there's got to be.... right? There's something that I always seem to come back to, a thought that always seems to be there no matter the train of thought. It's ever present with me and as today (12/07/2015) has gone on and the longer I've been off social media it's been growing.. 'I'm better off on my own' and do you know something, maybe I'm right, generally I do work better on my own because any thought process that I go through tend to get worked out better on my own. I don't want this to be taken as I don't want to be around people but I think for the next wee while I'll stick to my own company, I think it's better that way and to be honest it's something

I'm going to think about long-term, I need to be on my own for a bit, I think I get too involved with people and that's not where I need to be, plus taking myself off of social media is a good thing, I don't get on with it so you could say I've been proactive, you could but you probably won't. It doesn't matter, honestly. Am I depressive or is it that I just think at a deeper level than your average person, are the problems in my head medically related or are they caused by just how much I think? Obviously if I knew the answer to that I wouldn't be sitting writing trying to get to the bottom of it, I'd be sitting playing the xBox and not giving a toss about all of this, I only write when something is wrong and the fact that I've written nearly ten thousand words in less than five hours is giving me cause to think something isn't right or to put it more directly, it's making me think something is wrong. I said it earlier, looking back at my historic writing ninety five percent of it was when something wasn't right, all the little graphs I made and poems I wrote were all suggesting of something dark swirling through my head. All the previous writings pointed to feelings of despair, being unable to relate and a full-on assault against myself. Maybe I could run away, I mean... no-one would ever expect it. No-one would see it coming, obviously they would when you're reading this because basically it exposes the full detail of the plan but as I'm typing it it's definitely feasible. I need the silence of my own mind, I need quiet, I need lots and lots of quiet, there's too much goes on at my folks house in order for me to gather my thoughts, that sounds ungrateful but the longer this fight goes on the more I need to work out what I need in order to manage this, I've accepted I'll never beat this, that's fine, if I'm going to manage it though I'm going to need to surround myself with everything I need to get through this when it/he strikes. One thing I definitely need is my own space, I don't have that right now and I don't want this being taken as an excuse but I have been going out drinking, mainly because I need time to myself, it's one thing I desperately need right now and I just don't have it. God that sounds awful, I love my parents, I do and they are amazing. I just wish that I didn't have to deal with this. It's even harder to deal with when they're around, there are days I need to sit in silence, I don't have that option right now though. The more I'm writing the more I think I'm learning to understand what goes on in my mind, I've read my first two back and although they're insightful I don't think they hit what I need to hit. Don't get me wrong, I'm not knocking what I've written but when I read them back I just don't feel like I thought they'd make me feel when I read them. I'm proud, I'm proud of the journey that I'm going through and I've accepted that my goal in life is knowing I need to find effective ways to manage it. I think I've done ok, yea' there have been times where I've not managed it well but I'm not a machine, I'm human, as much as there's a lot that goes on inside my head I do a pretty good job of managing this, this isn't easy, this isn't something that I particularly like having to juggle but I do and the fact that I manage it is something I take great pride in. Just sometimes it gets really hard to deal with, those are the days that I would gladly trade. I'd quite happily take the flu for four days rather than go through what I have to go through, the depths I have to plumb, the amount of sludge and slurry I've got to trawl my mind through, the sheer mountain I have to climb just so I can get through the day and then get to my bed. Even then when I get to my bed what happens? I lay awake and I think, I get about four hours sleep and then it's time to face it all again. I can't even tell you just how hard it is to get up on days like that, my legs weigh ten tonnes, my head weighs ten tonnes and my mind weighs about twenty tonnes, ugh, it's on those days I wish I was simplistic, on those days I feel as if I would be best served locking myself in my bedroom and just not communicating with anyone, that's not being dramatic, that's actually what I feel like on those days, the word brutal doesn't even do it justice. I keep thinking about getting professional help, I mean it's never really something that's far away from the front of my mind but I don't know the best way to go about it, besides the fact I don't feel comfortable talking to my closest about the war that rages inside my head so how the heck am I going to talk to a complete stranger about it. I mean maybe I just need to take the plunge and do it, I've got material behind me now that helps but I don't know, I want to... I'm just so scared. (On a side note, ten thousand words and not one swear word, that's got to be the longest I've went without swearing) *I AM AN ALCOHOLIC* And I am, just writing it helps because I am. I don't drink to socialise, I drink to forget, I drink to escape and I drink just for the sake of drinking. It's a nasty thing to admit but I have to admit it, this is all about the truth and if I sit here and lie about it then I'm not going to get anywhere am I? I do use it as a coping mechanism and I do actually sometimes crave a pint. With a little resolve over the next couple of weeks I'm looking to reduce my alcohol intake as I need to focus on myself without booze, it does genuinely help me if done in moderation and I know it's a depressant, that's why I know if I drink in moderation then it does genuinely help me unwind, unfortunately though it's not always done in said manner and occasionally I do hit the bottle hard, I can't say I enjoy it much but I actually do it out of boredom a lot. As I stated earlier I get bored easily and it's just what I do, yes ok it's not ideal but it's something I need to manage, with me it's not really about enjoying life a lot of my time is spent managing the varying different things that go on in my life. God I feel as if I'm reflecting on my life thirty years too early, I'm reflecting and talking about regrets, jeezo I'm thirty-three, why the hell am I doing this? I'll tell you why I'm doing this is because I have to, I've said it before and I'll continually say it, I am not the same as your average person, my head does not operate as it 'should', it's something I'll say until I'm blue in the face, I won't apologise for it and I certainly won't shy away from it, I've spent way too long doing that, now's the time where I've got to face it head on. This is why I'm writing, this is why I'm delving, digging, unearthing, rearing, you name what I'm doing and I'm doing it. I want to get this all out so I don't need to write anymore, it's not even the fact that it hurts it's the fact that I'm missing out on so much because of my mind's inability to cope with the majority that it sees and feels, yet another thing I've always said is I feel my mind operates at a highly sensitised level, I feel a lot more, I feel compassion more, I feel empathy more and when all of that combines it unbalances me, it does it causes an imbalance in my head and that's what leads to the not so good days/the bad days and dare I say it, they lead to 'him'. I don't know if maybe I'm trying to fix something that's not broken or if I'm trying to fix something that's totally broken, this links back to what I was saying earlier, I just do not know what or how I feel, it's this big empty hole that just doesn't seem to be filled. I feel it, I feel things but it's almost like what's in my head over-rides the feeling if that makes sense? I feel, I genuinely feel but it gets numbed, it gets lost in the weight of my mind and then I don't know what I feel. It's hard, it shouldn't be this hard but it is. It's something I accept but it doesn't stop me from fighting it, it doesn't stop me wanting to be like everyone else and it will never stop me from trying to be like everyone else. Out of this I'm determined to live as normal a life as possible, I want to live my life and then die, I do not want to die and throw my life away... .....if only it was that simple. See, the fight and the hunger are there, the desire is there so I know I'm doing something right. I know deep inside this vault of a mind I've got it, I know it's there but I just need to unlock it, I need to fight through the weeds, the dirt and the mire to get to it. The good stuff's there, I've felt it before and I know it's there for me. I just need to find a way of getting to it and then keeping the bad stuff away from it. I don't use this line often but I deserve at least that much, I do, I've worked hard enough for it. I don't want to see hell or him again, quite honestly I've seen enough of both to last a lifetime, I don't need them anymore, I've seen the depths and the demons too much, I'm tired of seeing them, I'm focused on finding the good stuff again, the simple stuff, the nice stuff. The end of the working day and chilling with friends stuff. That's what I'm working towards, that's what I want from life, that's what I'm aspiring to, I want the simple things, I want the nice things. All I want are my friends, my family and the good times and as long as I'm breathing I'm going to fight for them. I need to fight for them because if I don't I'm not fighting for anything, I'm a man without a dream, a rudderless ship, a directionless wanderer destined to wander the rest of my life wondering, a 'what if' kind of guy, an 'if I'd only done this kind of guy', nobody wants to be that guy surely, I certainly don't. I want to do things, I want to travel the world, grow a big beard, get tattooed, spend quality time with friends and family, meet new people, become interesting. I want to do stuff, I want to see stuff, I mean that's not a lot to ask is it? I don't think it is to be fair. I mean it's achievable, I don't think what I've said there is the most ambitious set of life goals that anyone has set, I mean I'm never going to score the winning goal in a final or win the Nobel Peace Prize, I'm not being unrealistic here am I? In fact I think I'm being quite the opposite, I think I'm actually being quite realistic about the whole thing. It just comes down to being able to control my mind, that for me is the biggest challenge I face. Granted it's a pretty big challenge but definitely one I can win. What I'm trying to illustrate here is yes I'm not the biggest fan of my mind and yes I've got a lot to deal with but it doesn't stop me fighting and it doesn't stop me dreaming. I mean I've got to, I mean if I don't then what's the point of me actually being here, what's the point of me writing and what's the point of me trying. If I don't have a dream I don't have a reason to fight and if I stop fighting then we all know how that's going to turn out, I don't ask for much out of life, I don't want tonnes of money because if I do I'll be dead within a year, I don't want flashy cars because they just don't interest me in the slightest, I don't want fake friends because I'm not in high-school anymore and quite frankly those days are behind me. I don't really want anything out of life except my friends, my family and just that little bit of peace and quiet. A place where I can just be free from the mess that goes on inside my mind. I mean that's not too much to ask for is it. I mean I want the simplest of simplest things, it's just that he interferes and when he interferes I'm screwed, I mean I am absolutely screwed, he's interfered twice in my life and the twice he's interfered it's nearly cost me my life, I don't like being at the bottom of the ocean, I don't like the cold, I don't like being able to see my friends but yet not get near them, I don't like reaching when I know I'm too far away to touch them. I hate the galoshes,

I hate being trapped, I hate the feeling, the fear, the isolation and the pain. I hate the pain the most, I hate crying when I know that I'm trapped, I hate being trapped, I hate the fact that he is there laughing at me the whole time whilst I'm stuck there, I hate him laughing when I know it's him that's locked me there, I am his prisoner and until he says so I'm not moving, I am helpless, I am weak, fragile and at his mercy. I have no say, I have no power and worst of all I don't have the one thing that I need to face him, I don't have control. It's the control that's the worst, that and the cold, that and the fact that I know that I'm helpless to stop him, I know he can see me at the bottom, arms folded across my knees, staring helplessly, sobbing helplessly, sitting there at his beck and call, his mercy, it's his desire to keep me down that makes me want to get back up even more, I haven't named him, I refuse to name him, I'm happy leaving him as 'him', he'll always be 'he', it's bad enough when he comes to pay me a visit, it'd make me one hundred times worse if I named him, I don't want to name him, I don't want him in my life, why is he in my life, why does he want to put me there, why does he want to make me suffer? Why do I suffer? Why do I ache when this hits, why am I absolutely powerless to do anything about it? I pride myself on my ability to fight depression, it happens a lot more than people know. The fact that I fight it somedays without people knowing takes a lot of strength, it takes every single fibre of my being for me to do it but I do. I just get on with it and I do it. No-one asks for this, I certainly didn't, if it was up to me I'd stay as far away from this as possible, I hate it, it actually makes me want to vomit, I absolutely detest when it comes around, it's the cycle of it, the knowing that it's happening that's the worst. I touched on this earlier but that is by far the worst part of it, it makes me feel ill when I know it's coming. The blue sky is replaced with grey, the temperature drops and I feel the cold, I can manage but when I see that cliff and the water below then I know it's time to really brace myself, I know it's going to be ugly. How can I describe it accurately, can I describe it accurately? I don't know if I can. That's probably the best way I can surmise it. It's like someone reaches inside me and pulls every single emotion out of me apart from fear and even that gets numbed, the days where I feel nothing are by far the worst, they're a gut-wrench of a day, two days, three days, sometimes it lasts a week and then for no reason it disappears. It just ups and leaves me, it deserts me and leaves me wondering what happened, it leaves me asking why. I'm still asking why. It knocks me sideways. It's a total pain in the ass. (ass isn't swearing so it's not being counted as a swear...) Psychologically though it does take it's toll, I don't feel the same for days, even though I feel lighter when it lifts I never feel myself again until about two days later, maybe even three days later. It's like a fatigue, it is fatigue because mentally I have to fight, I need to constantly fight so I'm absolutely and completely shattered. Fifteen years this has been going on, fifteen years so obviously there are going to be scars, that much is obvious but what I don't understand is why, I don't get why I have to go through this, why I have to endure psychological warfare, what ultimately is the fight, what's the cause of it? I certainly don't know but what I do know is this. That first day when I've got to be around people and I'm in a state of silence is the worst, I want to talk, I want to tell people not to worry about me but at the same time I can't, my mind is in silence and therefore I cannot speak unless I have to and by I have to I mean anything work related, anything else is a short, brief conversation. My mind allows it but no more. I spend two or three days almost in a state of razor-sharp focus, I am so efficient at work because it's all I can do. My productivity soars because it's all my mind will allow me to do. Believe me I have wanted to force myself out the other side but I dare not try, that's stepping into the unknown and quite frankly it's bad enough dealing with the mental silence, never mind the possibility of adding more things on top of it, I just don't see that ending well. I'm sorry, I guess this is going a little bit deep, I am sorry if it's tough to read but believe me it's not much fun for me dealing with it, on my good days I am absolutely fantastic and on my bad days I'm just a wall of silence. The thing that annoys me the most by far are the good days that turn into bad days for no reason, the days where I'm coasting and then suddenly, 'BANG!' straight out of nowhere my mind capitulates, those are the days that I find hard to stomach, I don't deserve them, I don't think I deserve them, the bad days are bad enough, never mind having to have to unexpectedly deal with a bad day. They actually happen more than I'd like but thankfully they happen when I'm on my own so I can manage, when I'm out and they hit that's what I don't feel fair. When I'm out and I get hit he is the architect, I'm sure of it. He has to be otherwise why would it happen? I mean it's like a switch is flipped and that's it, I shut down and I have to leave, occasionally it's caused me to cry, this is walking through Glasgow by the way this isn't me on my own. I have to walk with my head up because in Glasgow I need to cross roads, on my own in the house is fine but I hate people seeing me cry. I'm pretty sure that's not normal, I think a lot of what I feel and experience is (relatively) normal but that isn't, that's not fair on me and certainly not on my friends who then worry. As I say I can take it, I'm a big boy I can take it on the chin but I don't think it's fair that my friends have to worry about me. That's not right and I don't like it one bit. Like all things though I just have to deal with it but then again that's what annoys me, even when I'm feeling close to my best I know I've always got to be on high-alert because I know somewhere in there it's lurking, prowling like a lion stalking a zebra, I know it's there because I feel it. Even on good days I'll be going about my business and just for a moment I know it's present, I can't see it, I can't pinpoint what's caused it but I damn sure know it's there. That right there is an annoyance, knowing that it's always somewhere in my mind, knowing it's watching and knowing it can strike me at any time, that's why I've got to always be extra vigilant. I don't want any surprises, I don't like when it comes out and surprises me, I can handle it on my own but when I'm with friends I can't, I have no time to prepare for it, I've got to just deal with it the best I can until I get home and then I can start to deal with it properly. I know what to do when I get home, I just don't like not having that level of control, I don't like being out of control and out of my mind at the same time, it makes me uncomfortable, it's too raw for me, it's like having my nerve endings exposed and the fear is touching them. It's painful, it's way too painful for me and it's too much to deal with me. It's when that strikes me I can sit and look out the window for hours, I can sit still for hours and focus on one flower, one tree, one car for hours at a time, I don't move, my hands stay clasped, my phone goes off and I don't respond, I don't even need to go to the toilet, I just sit, hands clasped looking, a blank stare across my face, my legs spread about two feet apart and all I do is stare, all I do is stare, I do nothing else, I just... sit. I'd love to say that after a few hours it goes away but it doesn't. That's the nice part of it, that's the good part of it. The bad part is when the thoughts start to swirl, the vortex opens and the hurricane starts heading towards me, I...am... powerless to stop it, I have no control over what it destroys, it just rips through my head like a hurricane through an old treehouse, nothing survives, it's best if I just lie there because if I try to fight it it just comes at me harder. I mean... it destroys everything, it takes everything I've built up and it just tears it apart like wet paper. I'm left with nothing again, I'm left there to go to sleep and just pick up the pieces, I mean I do, I start again, I have to start again because if I don't then my mood won't recover and I won't recover. I pick up the pieces because I believe that I'm strong, I have to believe in my strength and in my strength my belief is to build myself even stronger so when it comes again I'll have a better chance of my happiness staying intact. To my credit I am actually getting stronger and I do feel stronger but the big test is not when I'm feeling strong, it's when I'm at my weakest, THAT is the big test and then I have to see just how much I've built, I never outrun the vortex, there's no point trying because that happens, the big test is the hurricane that ensues, if I can come out of that with the foundations standing then I know I'm strong, I'm living in the belief that if I fight this battle long enough then eventually I'll be able to withstand the hurricane or maybe even the hurricane won't come my way. If the hurricane doesn't come my way then maybe I can avoid the vortex and if I avoid the vortex then maybe, just maybe I stand a chance of outrunning this and living my life as I see fit. That's the dream anyway, I don't know if that'll ever happen but I need to use the time I have to build again, I need to make use of this time so I can fortify, bolt and strengthen my mind because god knows when the next storm is coming, the last one I had was over a month ago so fingers crossed it's a long time before the next one hits. The dream is that another one doesn't hit but whether that happens or not we will just have to wait and see. Actually scrap that, I'll have to wait and see. Should life be this hard? The short answer, nope. Then again I can't imagine my life being any other way, I know that's going to sound a bit..... bleugh but I genuinely can't see my life being lived in any other mindset, I think the logical answer way of looking at it is because I know no other way. I'm just fascinated by people though, I people watch a lot when I'm commuting, I do the same walking to work, I guess I'm just naturally curious, I always have been it's my way. I just like observing people, I should have worked in science instead of going down the call centre route, I could have been the shiz at behavioural studies, it could have been my wheelhouse, I could have made something of it. Watching and talking to people all day about their mind and what's in it, I think I might have just had a 'mindgasm', yea' I know that's pretty schoolyard humour wise but I am genuinely intrigued by people, not just their mind but their wee quriks, mannerisms and idiosyncrasies, I love them all, I love watching them, from people sorting their lunch to people turning a paper, I like seeing how people dress as well, it's all just one big people watch that I'm on. To an extent I do it when I'm out as well, watching people's behaviours change as the alcohol takes hold, it's inevitable but the change is quite fun to watch, well I'll rephrase that I'll do it until I get tipsy and then I just end up getting drunk and stagger home, it won't be the first time I've people watched whilst drunk and it won't be the last time. I guess what I'm trying to say is even though I feel I'm different to most people I'm still in love with people and how each and every person has almost perfectly unique mannerisms and behaviours. I'm sad that way, I think you're reading this going, 'ha, loser'. You might not be but it fascinates me, I'm up at 5am tomorrow for work and I'll guarantee you I do it on the train to work tomorrow. I don't think I actually stop people watching, it's actually quite fun when you see the same people every day depending on what shift I'm on. For example there's one guy who gets the train from Glasgow Queen Street to Charing Cross, he always reads a book and he always turns the page quite aggressively, I stand next to him on the train and he doesn't know I watch him... but I do. People are fun, try it. I try and pick up what different people do, especially with newspapers, some lick their thumb then turn the page, other people feather the page over. It's the same with typing, some people WHACK the keyboard, others tap tap tap, some touchtype and some you just can't hear. The more I write this the more I realise I'm really interested in people, I've always tried to keep my distance from people, especially women because I'm scared that if I get into a relationship then I'll get hurt. Now I know that sounds soppy as hell but it's true, I'm phenomenally scared to get involved because I'd have to something I never ever do, let people in. The sheer thought of that terrifies me, can I let someone in? I don't know if I can, I mean I want to but jeez, could I open up and talk? Can I open up and talk? I'd actually quite like to do that because I know I encourage people to talk things out. I'm there for people so maybe it could work. I'm scared though, it's a big step to take. I guess I'll have to take that one as it comes eh? When I'm not people watching and I'm on the train I often sit and daydream out the window, I sit and I wonder what the future holds for me. I wonder what I'll be doing when I'm thirty four, the magical age of thirty five and beyond, what will I be like when I'm old? Where will I be career wise, where will I be staying? What will I actually look like in four years time, what will Glasgow look like, will I still be friends with the same people? I just sit and I ponder, I'll tell you one thing, it makes short work of the thirty minute commute from Larbert to Glasgow, it makes mincemeat of it. I get on the train and before I know it I'm in the tunnel at Queen Street although whenever I hit that tunnel I always fancy a nap, I have no idea why. It's the same when I have a few pints on my own, (not the nap part) I get lost in my own thoughts and I just tune out, before I know it fifteen minutes have past and I've finished my pint, I mean I completely and utterly tune out, it doesn't always happen but when it does it's quite nice, it's actually a really good place to be because it means I'm relaxed and when I'm relaxed I feel good, when I feel good... .. well you get the idea where that's going. Is any of this making sense? It makes sense to me because it's the inner workings of my head so I know what I'm saying, I don't know if it's translating across though, I hope it is because I want you to see what I see and feel what I feel through both good and bad. This for me is a journey, a journey that I didn't necessarily want to be on but one that regardless of how I feel I have to go through, sometimes there's beautiful sunshine, other times there are endless dark tunnels, I think it's too simplistic to say I've got to 'take the rough with the smooth', my journey's a lot more complicated than that and by the end of it I don't know what the outcome is going to be. I'd love to sit here and say that everything will be peachy but I know that's not true, I know ahead there are going to be really tough times and I know I'm going to need that build up of mental strength, god knows where I'm going to end up in terms of relationships. I mean I could end up getting married and having kids, well, not me having kids but you know what I mean with that. I mean that's something I've never even thought of, actually when I think about it there's a good reason that's never even entered my mind. I need to work on getting myself right first before I even consider entering a relationship and when I say 'getting myself right' I mean being in a position to be able to talk about anything that's not right i.e. bad days and the like. I mean for me it's hard to deal with never mind having someone else having to deal with it. I know if I meet the right person they'll love me regardless as I will with them but I'm not there just yet, maybe by the time I'm forty-three and all grey and the like. I don't know, I'm moving on though, that's definitely a worry/conversation for another day. For any of my friends/family reading this I know it's hard, it's hard me writing this, after the first two I thought this would get easier but it doesn't. You guys need to know that I give this one hundred per cent and I am in a much better place than what I was back in December. For anyone outside friends and family reading this I don't know what your opinion is but I hope it gives you an insight into just how fragile and breakable the human mind can be. In my case it's a fine line between strength and breakage, it's a combination of a three inch thick steel vault door and a flimsy wooden door. It's not intentional it's just the way I am and it's something I need to manage. Before I close this off I need to address 'him'. I don't know where he came from, I don't want to know where he came from but I'm trying so hard to control him. This is the first time I've actually been able to pinpoint exactly what I feel when the heaviness descends, I know somewhere I'm being watched and it scares me a little I'm not going to lie. Please believe me when I say I really don't like being so up and down, I mean I LOVE when I'm up and feeling great but doesn't everyone, it's just those days when he appears that I know I'm in trouble. Actually I've had enough of 'him', I don't want to think of it anymore tonight. For anyone that suffers with depression I'd ask you to reach out, it's by far the hardest thing you will ever have to do but it's totally worth it. You don't need to suffer in silence, it is by far the greatest mistake you can make, I'm talking from experience because for months I hid it and it nearly cost me my life, talk to someone, anyone about it. Call 'The Samaritans', phone someone, speak to a friend, the sooner you can talk about it the better you will feel. Although for me it was hard and I ended up crying I did eventually manage to talk to someone and I did feel better, I ended up with a great support network but I nearly left it too late, I waited way too late before asking for help. Please please please don't ever be afraid to ask for help, speak to your GP, they're there for you and will support you one hundred percent, go online and search mental health forums, talking online can be just as effective, I would encourage anyone reading this who has any mental health issue to seek advice when they can. It's not as easy as that, I know but there are people that care, your friends care and there are kind people out there who are by your side. You're not alone, never think that you are. That being said I know how it feels, I've used words like 'trapped' and 'abyss' and that's exactly what it feels like, it feels like an absolute hole you're down and there's no escaping, it is the absolute worst place to be and unless you speak to someone that understands they won't be able to help you. I count myself really lucky because my best friend went through the exact same thing at the exact same time and I couldn't have made it this far without her. She helped me so much when I was at my worst, she was there when I was walking about all the time with a pair of yellow sunglasses on all the time, they were my way of hiding, she's been there for me through thick and thin and I love her to bits, I've always counted myself really lucky because I somehow end up with amazing people in my life, I'm not really sure I deserve them but I'm glad I have them, I'm definitely a people person and I've been there for more than my fair share, I've laughed with friends, cried with friends, hung out with friends and got drunk with friends, if I had a choice between having a million pounds or my friends what would I choose? God the money, you wouldn't see me for dust! I kid, I'd choose my friends because they're loyal to me and I'm loyal to them, I am nothing without the right people in my life. I've denied this for years but I need people in my life, I need the banter, the conversations and the company, although I need time to myself I'll crumble if I don't have my friends, they are the ones who give me strength, they're the ones I know I can count on if I'm having a bad day, they're the ones that pick me up and carry me until I feel better and vice versa. Friends are a wonderful thing, people are a wonderful thing, never ever underestimate the awesomeness of people, you'd be surprised at just how awesome the right people are, they are fantastic human beings. I also have a fantastic family, I don't know where I'd be without their support, they have done so much for me and I am eternally grateful for all that they do for me, I've now learned that if I'm having a not so good time then I can talk to them, I know that they are behind me and talking to them isn't a sign of weakness, it's a sign of strength that I recognise that I can talk to them, I've said it before and I'll say it again, don't be afraid to talk to people that share the same fears as you, you might surprise yourself by what you find. Underneath all of this I am actually quite a simple guy, all I really want to do is the usual kind of stuff that a guy my age does, after work go and meet my friends, dance the night away in Rufus T Firefly/Solid Rock and listen to some good old fashioned rock and roll, I love music, I love going to gigs, I love my friends, I LOVE my friends, I ABSOLUTELY FRICKIN' ADORE MY FRIENDS, I am surrounded by great people, I'm surrounded by a great family and although they don't know half of what I actually go through they should know this. They mean the absolute world to me and I want them to know until the day I die I will love them ten thousand times more than they will ever love me. I want them to know that they are my world and without them my world is dark, without them I am forever locked in a basement with a blindfold on and no way of getting out, without them I do not have the strength to go on, I do not have a direction, without them I am well and truly fooked. Without everyone around me the world is a much darker and scarier place, without them I am nothing, with them I am everything, I fly, I soar and I believe, I breathe, I believe, I breathe and I believe. I am all that I can be with them behind me, they are my world, my rock and my strength. Without you I am merely a human, with you I can be me, with you my struggles have a light, without you I'm lost, floundering in the abyss, it's five hundred miles wide and I'm looking for a key, it's pitch black without you guys, with you beside me I am so much greater than what I am on my own. I feed off of your strength and your love, you're loving me propels me, it pushes me to be better, it pushes me to work harder, with you I am invincible, bulletproof and the definition of resiliency, without you I am unprotected and alone. I cannot live without you guys and if I don't have you guys... I cannot live, I am a flower starved of light and water, I will wither and die. I will disappear, wander and die. I will be mourned and forgotten, I will be a memory without you, I will always be with you but in spirit and mind, not in person. I need you, I am nothing without you, you guys are what drive me to beat this and I need you, I cannot do this without you, stay behind me, I need your strength for when mines fades. I love you, I don't say it enough but I love you more than I could ever speak or write, I love you unconditionally, I love you with faults, with anomalies, inconsistencies and flaws, I love you all and I always will. I just... find it hard to say that, it's what I feel, it's all I feel, I have so much love for everyone in my life but I can never say it. I want to say it but I just can't, it's not the done thing to just blurt out to someone that you love them. I don't want to disappear, I don't want to wither and die, I want to fight this again and I want to beat this, I want to enjoy myself and I want to be surrounded by the people I love the most, I know I'm not on my own with this, I know that but it's hard trying to open up with something you've been fighting on your own. The amount of times I have lay in bed crying over my inability to talk you wouldn't believe, the amount of times I have stared at myself in the mirror and tried to find something to believe in. I fight so hard and I fight all the time, I constantly fight this but it gets tiring, it gets so unbelievably tiring. That's why I need those around me, I need them for what lies ahead of me, for what I'm going to face. If I have my friends and family by my side then I have a chance, I NEED you a hell of a lot more than you will ever need me. You guys actually have no idea what you mean to me, I could write one hundred thousand words and I probably couldn't even scratch the surface of what you mean to me. I love you with all my heart and even though I'm inevitably going to have bad days, that doesn't mean that every day is going to be a bad day. Guys you need to understand that this cripples me, I mean emotionally and mentally it absolutely cripples me. I've been to hell, it's nothing special. Let's make a lifetime of memories and when we're all old and grey we can look back and laugh at all we went through. Let's make this the start of something beautiful.

October 2015

It never seems to leave me. I mean it's just always there and do you know the thing? I can't seem to think it, say it or write it without thinking I'm being dramatic. I can't even think about it without thinking there is actually nothing wrong with me. It started again today (12/10/2015) although in fairness I knew it was coming. I've been drinking a lot, I've been just all over the place, my temper has been short, I've been phenomenally short on patience and did I mention that I've been drinking a lot? I just don't feel like this is ever going to lift. I should be at the peak of my happiness the now, I should be king of the world, top of the world, basically any sort of happiness reference should be inserted here. ..but it's not. I just wish I knew how to deal with this, I wish I could do something constructive rather than what feels like 'mentally menstruate', that's the best way I can describe it, I apologise about that reference but I feel it's the best one to use. It's how it feels though. At this very moment I just feel like absolute fucking shit and there's nothing I can actually do about it. That's the thing that gets me about it. If there was something I could do I would do it... but I can't. I was sitting on the train tonight and I couldn't look straight ahead. I kept flicking between music, I kept screwing my face up, looking down, up, left right. It was like I was trying to replicate the original 'Sonic the Hedgehog' cheat using my face. (Up, Down, Left, Right, A + Start) I mean I just couldn't sit still, I think part of it was down to the fact that when I feel like this I don't want to hide any of it. I don't want to sit and look like everyone else, I don't want to play on my phone like anyone else, I don't want to look at anyone else... I am not everybody else and the sooner I realise that the better. I'm hurting just now and I could actually just sob, I could drop everything I'm doing just now and sob. I could cry my eyes out, maybe that'll make me feel better? So I know what the general reaction to this is and I know what the thinking is going to be when I say it but I don't care, I'm going to say it anyways... .. I need alcohol. Yes, I know it's a depressant, yes I know it doesn't help but with me it does. I spend a lot of my time searching, I spend a great deal of my time searching actually. I don't know who I am, I'll freely admit this, I don't know where I'm going in life or what I actually want to achieve. I don't know whether to laugh or cry, if I'm seen as bold or a dumbass. I don't know what people see of me, I don't know what my parents see of me and I sure as hell don't know what I see of me. It absolutely tears me into lots of tiny pieces, I accept it though because that's the way I'm wired. I accept it and I deal with it but today.. ugh today I can't accept it because as well as pondering what my life means to me and who I am and who I want to be and the nine million other thoughts in my head I've got the super fun time of my mind racing to deal with. Happy.. fucking days. I mean happy days. So as well as having an already bursting mind I've also got the fun of my mind in warp drive mode, brilliant. Absolutely fucking top class, I could not be any happier right now. I mean... as well as managing everything else I've got going on let's add more things on to it because more always helps right? No, not right. Wrong, fucking... wrong. It's all fucking wrong right now and I'll admit that. The question is the same as it always is. 'What's causing it'? Maybe nothing is causing it, maybe it's the fact that we're in the process of changing from season to season. Maybe it's the fact it's getting dark quicker now, maybe it's because I've been under a lot of stress the last few weeks or maybe it's down to the fact that my sheer hatred of people and my inability to work them out is coming to the surface. There, I said it. Yea', I do hate people, I have a lot of great people in my life but generally I do have a lot of hate for them. I particularly hate 'gameshow people'. You know the ones, the ones that know an answer but because they know it they'll milk the fucking cunt right out of the fucking thing. Oh god I hate that, why can't you just answer it? Why can't you just pick A,B or heaven forfend even fucking C? Why do you have to kick the arse out of it and make yourself look like a first class fucking idiot. I apologise about the language but it's going to be a recurring thing so I'm afraid you'll need to adjust. I swear a lot at the best of times, never mind when I'm mentally down and I'm ranting. So, apologies but, it's going to happen. Do you want to know what I often think of? I often think about running away. Maybe I could, I don't think people care as much for me as they say they do. Often I feel like I'm a convenience in people's lives and I'm there when I'm needed for advice or something. Now I might be well off the mark with this but it's something that's been nagging me for the last couple of months. I just feel that maybe I'm not cut out for this 21st century living stuff; maybe I'm not cut out for social media, smartphones and civilisation. I don't think social media and me mix when I feel like this. I need to stay off it because it's at times like these everything really irritates me. The thing is though, generally everything does irritate me, I am a misanthrope. Maybe it's about time I accepted it. Maybe if I accept I hate people and stop faking interest in people I'll feel better? Maybe if I just act like myself then I'll feel better. Maybe I could do everything I should and I'll never feel better? At the moment that's what feels like the most plausible theory. So this question is going to crop up repeatedly again but once again, I guess you'll just need to adjust. 'Do you know something'? So, do you know something? I don't even know why I'm typing this up, I mean what am I actually looking to achieve out of it? I've written three before and all that it's done is given me a temporary lift. I mean all of that just for a temporary release? Great. So at least I can stop lying to myself and say that I write because it makes me feel better because it fucking doesn't and why should it? There's no reason that me tearing myself apart should make me feel better. It should do the exact opposite and it should make me question what the fuck I am doing. What the fuck am I doing? And the answer is... I don't know. Like with ninety percent of things in my head I just don't know and that's one of the things that rankles me, it's one of those things that just eats away at me and slowly turns all the good to hate. I don't know if I need to be louder or quieter, I don't know if I talk too much or not enough. I debate my own dress sense constantly and something I've touched on previously in prior works, I analyse every single thing I say. Maybe it is actually best if I ditch the smartphone, the social media accounts and all the chat services and just go native. Get an old phone and use it for calls & texts and that's it. Do I need to know what everyone is up to at all times and vice versa? No, probably not. Do I have the resolve and the conviction to follow through with such an idea? No, absolutely not. I come up with all of these good ideas but I never follow them through. That's a huge failing of mines, once again something I'm really honest with and happy to admit, I'm good at admitting my failings, I just need to be better at following them up. I'm crap at following them up. Actually I'm not very good at doing anything and I'm not saying this in an attempt to get people to kiss my ass and make me feel better. I'm saying it as I genuinely believe I'm actually not really good at anything. I'm an average gamer, worker, snooker player, friend. I don't really have anything I excel at, nothing I can say 'Do you know what? I'm really fucking good at this'. Well actually.. that's not true because I'm really good at these: • Tearing myself apart • Upsetting myself • Over-analysing • Over-thinking So yea' actually I am really good at things but unfortunately nothing that's going to do anything positive for me. Ugh didn't think I could make myself feel much worse but I've just managed to do that very thing. Congratulations Dave you fucking tit. Maybe it's time to go back to the docs, maybe it's time that I just cut everyone out of what's happening, maybe it's time for me to start heading down to the basement again and start fighting all over again. I can't take this, I mean I can't... physically or mentally take this shit. I've got a work life to balance and adding this on top is like adding one too many bricks on Jenga, ugh. I just don't feel right just now, once again though I know I've not been feeling right again and it's not just because of the increase in alcohol and the mood swings, this time I've just been feeling detached from everything, this is a new thing before the depression has hit. This has been an altogether new experience and it's not necessarily a bad thing. Let me explain: I'm pretty intense, I'm exactly what you'd expect in a Scotsman, I'm angry, fiery, a nationalist and a big drinker. I would say it's a pretty fair statement to say I never switch off and I don't. I'm always fired up, ready, alert etc. Even when I drink I find it hard to shut off because my mind is always ticking, it's always thinking of things and I'm working in tandem with it trying to analyse what it throws at me. I'm a deep, deep person, I think I hide it well in social circles & work but when I'm alone I do analyse things and think. What do I think about? Basically, the above plus nine trillion other things at any one time, it's no wonder my head is fucked. Is it fucked though? It's definitely fair to say that what I experience isn't normal but is my mind fucked? No, I don't think so. I think saying that is a dramatization and this is being written in fact, not blown up by ridiculously big exaggerations. Is that what my head does? Does it take things and just blow them out of proportion? I don't know, maybe? It comes back to that ever recurring statement though... 'I don't know'. The thing is, I don't though and it bugs me. I'm thirty-three, thirty-four in general and I feel like my life is going absolutely fucking nowhere. I'm back with my folks temporarily and I don't want to be around them and I don't want to be on my own. I never ever want to be the place where I'm at and that isn't an exaggeration that is one hundred percent fact. When I'm at work I look forward to going home, when I'm at home I look forward to going to bed, when I'm in bed I look forward to getting up, when I.. ..I mean you get the idea right but I'm never comfortable in the place where I am, that slightly concerns me. I'm probably at my happiest when I'm at work because I've got tasks to focus on, my mind's got to be focused on the job in hand and that's fine. I can handle that, I like that, it's one of the few things I do like. The problems start when I'm outside of work because I'm lost, I nomad my way around my hometown, normally bouncing between pubs and writing. It's just my way and I accept that. I know this has started with a lot of swearing and vibes of I hate myself but I normally manage this pretty well, it's just the times I can't manage it the bad stuff goes down. I'll be frank and upfront right now. I don't really know where I'm going with this and I don't know what's going to come out so you'll need to bear with me. I don't know right now what I'm thinking, well that's a lie actually because there's quite a lot going on that I conscious of. The dislike of social media is one, the (general) dislike of people is another and this is one thing that I've definitely been thinking lately, I wrote it down last week and it's something I can't seem to shake. I was in one of my local pubs in Falkirk having a pint and writing as I do. Nothing was forthcoming so I had another pint and then I checked my phone, I kept getting messages so I kept pulling my phone out and replying (as you do). It was only then I looked round and realised that I'm tied to my phone. I was pausing my writing to use my phone and since then I've been looking around and seen other people tied to their phone, tied to social media and tied to whatever app they're looking at. I wrote something interesting and something I wasn't expecting. I wrote 'I am clone 15011982'. Now 15011982 is just my birthday but I feel that I am just another insignificant member of the smartphone generation, I am a part of 'Generation Why', generation smartphone, generation app, generation anti-social and the more I think about it, the more I wretch inside. The more I hate myself for being a part of it. I hate the fact I can now sit on my phone in a social environment, use my phone and it's now considered socially acceptable. It's not socially acceptable, it's downright fucking rude is what it is. The thing is though and I know it's going to happen is this'll pass and I'll just go back to being tied to my phone. Why should I be though? It's just not right and it doesn't sit well with me. I need to do something about it but as always I won't, I NEVER follow-up on anything. When I'm in this state I have really good ideas, I know this sounds like a contradiction but when I feel like this I do actually have some really good ideas and clear thinking. I mean granted it doesn't happen often but sometimes everything calms and I can see things the way I want to. So going back to this jotting down about me being 'clone 15011982'. Am I? Are we all just different versions of ourselves? I feel like I am, I feel I'm just average guy #3 with the build of baggy trousers with chains, a shaved head and a horseshoe moustache. Am I any different to guy #4 with his trendy clothing and in-trend hairstyle? No. We're one and the same. The only thing that differs is guy #4 has a lot trendier clothing on, less of a belly than me and probably gets more sex in one week than I do in three years. That aside are we all different? No. (Obviously this is all opinion, just more of the crap that goes on inside when I'm out having drinks.) It's just this never ending soul-searching that mystifies me. I don't even know why I keep doing it because I don't really know what I'm searching for. Is it tranquillity? Is it stability? Is it just that little bit of sanity that staves away the demons? Once again, I don't know. It drives me absolutely fucking nuts because it goes from thinking to obsession, I can lose hours thinking and when you really break it down it's really hours thinking about absolutely fucking nothing. I mean, is this going to be me when I'm in my sixties and seventies, is there something drastic that's going to change in the next thirty-years? Am I even going to be here in two years? If you were to ask me that question could I give you an honest answer? No, I couldn't because I actually don't know and that's one of the times where I'm quite happy to say that I don't know. Since we're there I'd be as well addressing it. Suicide is still a frequent thought in my head, it's maybe not as prominent or as strong as it was but it's still there just running in the background, I see it and I know it's still present, I deal with it, it's fine but it's something that carries relevance. It all comes back to how I feel in society and the thoughts over the last couple of months have been along the lines of wanting to exclude myself completely from social circles. Granted I've not said anything but how do you say something like that? There's no easy way to say to people, especially people I'm close to that I want nothing to do with anything anymore. That's how I feel and I think that's the first time since I started writing it's the first honest thing I've managed to dig out from inside of me, I'll say it again just so I can affirm it: 'I want nothing to do with anything anymore'. Yip. It's true, the more I analyse it and the more I read it the more I want to do it and the more I want to do it. I don't do drama and situations well, I never have. It's one of the three thousand and sixty-five reasons I'm presently single. I just don't do drama and arguments and all that shit, I've got enough on my plate without worrying about a girlfriend who most likely will drive me up the fucking wall and vice-versa. Actually, I'm quite happy being single because not only can I do what I want when I want it also means when this strikes I can shut myself off from everyone and deal with it. Could I do that in a relationship? Hmm probably not, I think I'd find that hard. In fact scrap that, I think it'd be a nightmare so yea', happy to be single. What is this? I mean what is causing this? Is it imbalance, is it the change in season? Stress? Change in season is plausible and I don't want to over-look the fact that this time last year is when I had my worst ever struggle with depression, that's definitely a factor I do not want to over-look. It doesn't make it any easier though, it doesn't make it easier to manage/deal with. Social media isn't helping, whilst typing this up I'm thinking about ways to disengage social media and leave my friends validated because let's face it. Why should I think of myself, I mean, there's nothing wrong with me right? It's me throwing a bit of a moody, toys out the pram right? WRONG. The sooner I start accepting that me & social media don't get on the better. I'm not built for cat updates/checkins/baby pics and various tripe motivational quotes. If I'm being frank and honest I bore myself with social media updates so god knows what my friends & virtual friends think. The thing is though right, I'm going to do it and that's fine because I feel like total shit the now. I know I do and I've got to work through this. The good thing is I know I'll work through it and that's fine. The thing that annoys me though is when I feel better I'll want to go back on it, why though? Why do I want to go back on social media? Boredom? Obsession? OCD? I don't fucking know but I'm looking at it right now (12/10/2015) and it's just fucking shit. I can see a baby on my feed and yet another witty, funny meme shared between friends. Do you know what social media is? In-jokes, tonnes and tonnes of injokes intertwined between various feeds. God I actually hate it, I'm actually feeling this is therapy, you know the classic phrase 'Let it out', well this is me letting it out so here goes... *deep breath & 1...2....3'. This all started with something that I couldn't shake from about four, five years ago, it was when I first went through my first real battle with depression and it's stuck with me ever since. 'I was born in the right mind but born at the wrong time'. Yip, I actually agree with that and the writings I jotted down confirmed that, I looked back at them frequently and most things came back to that exact thought process. I wish I was the age I am now but in the sixties, seventies or eighties. I embrace technology but my head can't cope with the sheer amount of data and endless pointless arguments. I think too much at the best of times so when I see various postings/arguments/links/memes/baby pics/cat pics/food pics/arguments/arguments/FUCKING GOD DAMN ARGUMENTS my head just.. can't handle it, it doesn't accept it, it rejects it and quite right. Do I need to know where people are checking in, what they're up to, what their cat or pet is doing and likewise. No, the answer thankfully is a resounding, confident, over-whelming no. I check social media out of sheer boredom and for what? What is the big deal with it? I need to log out of social media and log in to what my head is actually telling me, that might be a fucking start. In fact, that IS a start. Now I'm not trying to get across that I'm holier than thou and fucking perfect in social media, I'm not and I know I'm not but it all ties in with how I've been feeling the last few months and that links back to the whole 'I feel like a convenience', social media just helps me affirm that fact. I need a break from it, I need to come off of it or the breakdown that ensues will be epic. I'm not ready for that, there's too much on my plate just now for me to have an epic breakdown. I've got things to manage but one-hundred social media and me need to split up. Why should I constantly feel like what I've put above and continue to go on it, it does nothing for me so if I feel like I do and I'm on social media is this going to make me feel any better? No. Is it going to lift me? No. It's going to have the exact opposite effect, social media to me is what alcohol is to other people who suffer with depression and that is a depressant. If you can use it right then I guess it's great but for people that can't use it right or cope with it well, it needs to go so goodbye social media. I'm not confident but I hope I never ever see you again. Suicide. So, there it is. Let's just bring it right into play so there's no pussy-footing around it. It's there, it's in my head so be as well getting it down so I can look at it. So what am I seeing when I look at it? I see nothing; I look at it as if I'd just written the word 'socks' or 'coffee', no big deal. It's a thought isn't it? This thought used to terrify me, it would cause me to cry but now it just sits there like the ten million other things and it has no effect. I keep going back to it and looking at it, yip, absolutely nothing. I don't feel good just now, I mean I think I've maybe mentioned/conveyed that over the previous pages but just in case there's any doubt, I'm not feeling good but even when I feel good suicide still floats around my head, it's just always there, sometimes in the background, sometimes right at the very back of my head and sometimes it pops in there just for no reason. The good thing, in fact the important thing is the fact that it is never ever at the front of my head. If it's at the front of my head then yea', I know things are serious. The thing that would worry anyone else with this is I think it's something that will happen someday and I hope you appreciate that I am being completely honest here. I just don't see myself getting old, I see myself committing suicide and I'm not ashamed to admit it, I think there will come a day when I've fought and fought and I just can't fight anymore. I hope I'm wrong of course but no-one knows my mind like I do and no-one knows their mind better than the person that's living inside of it. I've thought about it, analysed it, assessed it and then over-analysed it but yea', I think maybe sometime about mid-forties? It's just something I can't shake and I'm glad that I can't because I think it's healthy. Here's the reasoning: I have been very lucky so far in life where I've not really had any tragedy, obviously I've had sadness but I've not had a totally catastrophic death that's thrown me miles off-course, I know I've still to have that but here's the thing about that, I'm prepared for it. I have to be. I cannot allow myself to be caught off-guard with a death and when I say a catastrophic death I mean a family member. I've built up my mind for it as I need to be ready for it happening, that is going to sound incredibly morbid but I need to do what's right for me. I need to prepare myself for burials/cremation, grieving and mourning and although it's not a nice subject I need to think about long-term mental health. On the flip side though, my death may come first because day-to-day I just need to evaluate this and deal with it. I still believe that it's going to be an achievement to go past thirty-five. That's still there and that's still ever present in my head, floating around there with organisation, planning for my day and suicide. These thoughts are normal, they're not normal to everyone else but they are normal to me. Considering all that goes on in my head I think I do pretty fucking well to manage my head, of course I'm going to have days like this, depression's a bitch like that. It strikes when we don't expect it, that's the nature of the beast and that's the reasons why the demons are so hard to face at times. They catch you cold. I'm lucky I generally know, I generally get a feeling so I can stick the walls up and curl up, ready to brace, face and deal with them. I don't know if that's common but do you know the thing is? I don't really care. It helps me and in times like this when I feel trapped in my own mind I have to do whatever it takes to power through the wall on the other side. It's just... it's that whole time when I'm stuck between the walls (i.e. now) that just absolutely sucks. It's just a never-ending cycle of regret, pain and being lost. It eats at me, takes chunks out of me, ruins any good thought/intention I have and most importantly/annoyingly of all it causes me just to block everyone out. The good thing is I'm learning to accept that though, as I'm getting older I'm definitely getting better at dealing with it, my mental stamina is getting better and generally people don't actually know when I'm suffering. I say generally and that's because when I'm suffering I now say to people openly. Like tonight when I came into work I got asked how I was. Honestly guys? Yea' not good and the words used were 'I know something's wrong', people respect that and I appreciate it. Tonight it's just a case of doing whatever gets me through my shift, I need that approach. My head is single-tracked tonight, the only thing I focus on is getting to seven am so I can go home and sleep. Don't get me wrong, I know I manage this well and I don't want a picture painting misery. I take a lot of comfort in just how strong I am and for all that goes on yea', I'm fucking proud of myself and how I take hits and keep on running. The part I dread the most is being in any social environment, at times like this I need my bed, a notepad and a cup of tea. I don't care for anyone or anything else right now; my sole focus is on me, myself and I. I was on the train to work and I just didn't handle it well. I just wanted to bury my head in my hands and cry, there were so many people, there were so many people laughing, checking their phones. The only thing I could take comfort in was the fact the sun was setting and the world was pretty through my yellow shades, they've been through a lot with me and for this fight I'm going to need them again. When I have them on I feel invisible, detached, stealth. I need them actually otherwise I'd be a mess. I've had them for a year and they've seen me at my worst, they're like battle-scars and the reason I go to them is because they give me strength. They're not pretty but I don't care, as I say whatever it takes to get me through. In times like this and I know this is going to sound silly but I need them, they're necessary. They're up there with the need to be alone, my bed, my notepad and my tea. They're vital. Maybe it's best if I just cut ties with everyone, so I can truly deal with this on my own, I just can't shake this whole feeling of being a convenience in my friends lives. Once again it's something that started as a nagging thought at the back of my mind and it's been pushing its way forward ever since. Maybe that's the direction I need to go? Ugh I digress. Wanna know where I feel I'm at the now? No, well I'm going to tell you anyways. I feel like I'm in the middle of fucking nowhere, it's pitch black and I'm bang in the middle of ten million junctions, that's where I feel I am and it's somewhere I get tired of being. Maybe it would be better if I just disappeared, started again. Maybe it'd be better if I just started again, moved somewhere new and just forgot everything about everything I've ever known. Maybe it's better if I'm dead? Maybe that'll finally quench the burning deep inside my soul. I mean what the fuck is it going to take? Keep bearing my soul every four or five months for temporary release? Is that what I'm striving for, is that what my release is? That's my crumb of comfort? Wow well fucking sign me up and hold me back. Anything has to be better than this; anything has to be better than feigning interest in things and people. Feigning interest in stories and fake laughing, acting like I care, acting like I give a fuck when really I don't. I genuinely don't give a fuck but rather than me following my convictions I talk myself out of it. This is making me sound ungrateful to everyone that's stood by me, it's not. I am grateful. In fact who am I even talking to, none of my 'friends' are going to read this! Haha that's amazing! It's taken me over five thousand words to realise that I'm ranting against myself, fucking brilliant Dave you first class cunt. Honest to fuck see whatever the opposite of The Turner Prize is you would definitely be in the running for it. I need some time away from people, the way this is going this isn't going to end well. As I'm typing this my hatred is growing but I look calm. I am calm I just…. I just get annoyed by too much, I get annoyed by commentators saying obvious statements, I get annoyed by people stating the obvious, like weather forecasters pointing out at this point in time (12/10/2015) that it's getting colder in the UK and Australia are seeing temperatures up to twenty-nine degrees fahrenheit. Well… obviously, we're coming into winter and they're edging towards summer so yea', there is a chance that our weather is going to get colder and theirs is going to get warmer. It's like when I'm watching golf and they interview the guy or girl that's one and the first question they ask is 'How do you feel'? How do you think they feel you fucking dumbass, they've just WON the very event they've just entered. You don't walk up to someone after a funeral and ask them how they're feeling so why the fuck are you asking someone that's just won something how they feel. You fucking fuckturd. See? That stuff drives me up the fucking wall. I HATE idiocy and stupidity, definitely two of my pet peeves, once again why being a part of 'Generation Fucking Why' grinds my gears. It's way too accessible for people to be idiots and stupid. You just need to log on to our good friend social media to see why. I'm going to go back so bear with me again but there is a point and I'll start with four words.. 'The Scottish Independence Referendum'. This... drove... me... nuts. Now before I start I'd like to point out I am a proud Scot and I voted Yes BUT I didn't do it blindly, I sat and deliberated for months about it, I wanted to vote Yes but only if I thought it was sustainable and the right thing for our wee country. Anyway I voted Yes and we somehow voted No, I'm not getting into politics because I need to feel better, not worse. Social media was an absolute fucking nightmare and I mean from July until the actual voting day it was chaos, I didn't know so many idiots existed, the arguments ranged from oil to culture even to personal differences! I mean it was fucking nuts and I hated being part of it. People fell out, harsh words were exchanged, digital friendships were thrown away and of course people of two certain big football clubs in Scotland had their usual unique, well thought out inputs. My point is this, everyone is entitled to an opinion, that's granted but what my head can't process is people throwing completely illogical arguments about, people that make really stupid points or the worst, people that actually don't know what the fuck they're talking about. I loved the independence referendum, I genuinely enjoyed watching the televised debates, I like debates as long as they remain somewhat factual. People who have access to social media have a free reign to do what they want and it's just a shame that a really good chance for lively debate turned into a mud-slinging match with digital ramifications. Anyway, we voted no and that's the end of it. Enough on it because it's starting to boil my blood, moving swiftly on. On the plus side it at least pulled me away from my head for a wee bit and to be honest I feel a wee bit better for it, whether I'll feel better at seven o'clock tomorrow morning is a different story.It just irritates me, I just don't know if I want to be facing this the rest of my life, I mean, suicide is the last option for so many reasons but will it actually quell my pain? I've attempted it once but I tapped out. I had the balls to do it and I should have seen it through, that statement is deliberate. If I'm going to do something like that then it's not fair to have so many people suffer. If it ever comes to it again, there is no tapping out, let's get that fucking clear. If the day comes where my reasons for dying outweigh my reasons for living then I need to involve no-one. That statement should be sending chills down my spine but it doesn't. It's like the word suicide it just.. sits there, as if I'm reading a junk email, it just does absolutely nothing. Maybe I'm more ill than I thought? Well there's nothing I can do about it tonight so it'll just have to sit there. I'm a mess mentally, I don't actually know if I'm coming or going, I don't know if I want to live or die and I don't know if I want to beat this or I want this to beat me. Once again, all sounds very dramatic but this is what's going on. I got a tattoo about a month ago, actually I got two. I got a semi-colon tattooed on my neck to symbolise like the sentence, the fight isn't over and a chest piece that reads 'The Devil & God Rage inside me'. Well, they do basically because I'm always caught between good and evil basically. It's where I constantly seem to be stuck between. I mean. Is it worth me looking at me getting help for something I may not actually want to get help on? I'm not sure. Sure I can go to the docs and bounce ideas off of him. Sure I can make these grand ideas up and I can formulate plans to deal with it but ultimately this is inside of me and it doesn't appear to be getting better. Maybe I don't want it to get better? Maybe me writing this is going to allow me to be honest and say 'I don't want to beat it'. Maybe... The more I read that back the more I can't decipher, I don't actually know if I want to or if I have the desire to do so. I feel inferior to people, I just don't feel I have anything to offer society, whether that's to do with how I feel just now or whether that's long-term I don't know. I mean that thought has been there for a while so that's definitely one I'm debating. I'm sitting just... thinking. I'm just sitting, scratching thoughts against the wall, desperately hoping one sticks there, endlessly looking down avenues for that one breakthrough that'll free me from this, that one thought or mantra that will relieve me of all this weight that's pushing my head down. I've got to. I have to. I NEED... to. If I don't do that then what chance do I have? I'm beginning to feel like this is hopeless, it's maybe not but all I can think of is removing myself from society, removing myself from friends and just leaving family and even then not letting them in. I want to run. Fight or flight is causing my hands to run cold, the blood is going to the legs prepping me to sprint away. Is that the answer? Cutting ties and just disappearing? It's definitely in there and it's stronger than suicide or any other thought I have. Do I plan it or just do it? How do I go about it? I mean I can actually feel the weight pushing my head down, my shoulders actually ache, weirdly the right one aches more than the left one but right on top of my head it feels like a weight is pushing it down, the back of my eyes hurt and my chest actually feels heavy. There's got to be something that causes this, I can't just be 'imbalanced', it's got to be more than chemical, there's something that causes this I'm sure of it. Yes I get warning signs, yes I'm grateful for them but what I'm not grateful for is how much this throws me, I'm beginning to think that there's no hope.

I'm beginning to wonder if people can forgive me. Forgive me for what I don't fucking know but if it comes to it.. would they forgive me? And here we are, back at those three fucking words.. I… DON'T… KNOW…… …and I don't, that's the thing. I've volunteered for a local mentalhealth charity where I stay, I done that on Wednesday of last week (07/10/2015) and I'll be honest I'm nervous. Can I handle that? Could I do it? I mean writing isn't doing it and apparently writing is very cathartic, well I'm sorry to say but it's not been fucking cathartic for me. I continually slice myself open only for the scars to heal and then bleed when it fucking well likes. Uch the more I'm writing the worse I'm feeling, it's like I'm pulling at this wound and nothing's there, it's phantom, it feels like it's there but it's not. But I feel pain so surely where pain is there has to be something there? I mean that's not far-fetched thinking is it? That's logic? Surely? Can someone please help me, I'm floundering, grasping at straws looking for anything that's going to see me through this. I need to get through this. Maybe if I go on social media…….. Aye, right who am I kidding, that'll make me feel better. I'd rather stick my head in a shredder than go back to that. My thoughts are all clashing against each other now, they're all trying to run through the same door and they're clashing, they're blocking everything so now I'm sitting trying to get some peace of mind and I'm getting static. There's nothing, there's no respite available. I'm in the worst place possible now and that's where my thoughts are racing and crashing against one another. It renders me useless, helpless and in safe mode. My mind is now entering the stage where I can't function unless the action ahead meets very strict parameters, this is the part of the depression I hate the most because I have nowhere to go, no shelter it's just like touching a raw nerve or an electric fence with the voltage full. Nothing works, nothing gives me that relief and it fucking sucks. Let me be clear, depression is a first class cunt to deal with, I don't use that word often and I am aware I've used it in this writing but it's not a word I throw about when talking about depression but I'm beginning to feel like I'm never going to beat this. It keeps coming back to that train of thought and it'll always come back to that. I'm sick of this whole thing, I know that's fairly generic but it's true. I do hate it. I hate the fact I'm now looking at the possibility of ostracizing people just to appease myself. It makes me sad. I don't ask for much, I'm a casual gamer, I like playing snooker, I like basically hanging out with people but will I ever beat this? One of those questions that makes me feel like I'm a pre-teen that's just broken up with his 'childhood sweetheart. Do you know what fuck that? Why should I constantly feel like I'm the one that's wrong and doing things wrong? I'm not doing things wrong, I'm doing things RIGHT and I STILL FEEL AS IF I'M

FUCKING WRONG. How is that possible? I'm not doing anything wrong,

even at one of my lowest ebbs I'm still refusing to acknowledge that I'm

not choosing this, I am not choosing to feel this way and I am most

certainly not looking at suicide for the sheer fucking fun of it, let me be

clear on that in case it wasn't. This is hard, this is very fucking hard, I'm

bleeding my guts out here and I'm the one that feels wrong? Why? Why

the fuck why??? That's not fair. That's not fair on me. This is serious

fucking shit, this unhinges me and takes me away from those I love, those

that stand by me and fight with me. I know I keep going over this but why

in the time that I need people do I feel that this is some big weakness? It's

not. It's perfectly acceptable, it's how I've trained my mind over the last

nine months, ever since I attempted suicide in December last year it's

what I said I would do and I've fucking done it. I've blew this open, I've

written about it, I've been open about it and I've fucking dealt with it. I

am dealing with it, this isn't fair. This is an affliction, a disability, a disease

but here I am working through it, no-one knows I feel this way so I just..

sit in silence? Is that the way I go about it? Aye because if I do that it's

going to end well isn't it? I have made such an effort to blow this open

and here I am belittling myself for it. Way to go Dave, that's really healthy doing that. I don't even know what I want now, (ha! As if I did before!) I don't know what my plan of attack is, where I'm going to go and how I'm going to fucking well deal with this. (I am trying to clean up the language but I'm emotive, what can I say. I am trying though….) I'm sitting here, it's just turned midnight and what am I doing? Trying to think, I just will not switch off. I drive myself crazy and the thing is I think I need to. I think I need to drive myself crazy. Bizarre statement? Well no not really. I like to think that by going through this it drags up a lot of the crap, kinda similar to a car running really low on petrol so it brings all the dregs of the tank up. Whereas that's not good for the car it's good for my head, I need this every once in a while but that's not to say I like it any better. I don't, I fucking hate it. I fucking hate everything right now and once again my conversations have hit a wall on social media, I swear to god I could scream just now. I don't mind conversations breaking down but three lines in I just don't get it. Am I that boring? Am I that uninteresting? Maybe I should get a tattoo across the front of my head that says 'Regular'. Would that help everyone? Would maybe fucking help me to accept that I'm just not that interesting, well according to the digital world anyways. So if the above is correct I'm writing this for the sake of my sanity. Well, maybe that's not a bad thing, it's the one thing I feel that makes sense and it's the one thing I'm barely clinging on to. Let's be honest if I don't have my sanity this thing is over, I mean if the sanity goes everything goes with it so saving that is definitely worth fighting for. At the moment though it feels about all that I can fight for? It's tough. It's hard to accept that I am this way, I keep hoping that one day this'll dissipate and I'll get myself back permanently. It feels just now I am a chameleon version of myself, depending on what social circle I'm in adapting to the needs and character of that group. That just tells me that I need to do one of two things, I either need to: • Be myself (*sniggers*, yea' right) • Gradually move away from my social circles. Option two is definitely more plausible than option one, I find it very very hard to be myself unless I'm on my own. If I'm around any single one of my friends I adapt myself to their character needs. I dare not speak my own mind, I stick to a certain formula that caters to said friend. That's horrifying, I'm reading that back and I actually do that, ugh it makes me sick that I actually do that. I need a lot of time myself, I need a LOT of time to myself, mainly because people drive me crazy, I may have mentioned that once or twice? The main reason I need a lot of time to myself is I need to process all that goes on, process, manage and then deal with it. Maybe I should spend more time on my own? Maybe that's the answer? Maybe I should just deal with whatever comes into my head on my own instead of letting it manifest itself and poison my view of others. If I don't have the others then the worst I can do is poison myself and let's face it, considering how hard this hits it wouldn't damage me that much. This is ridiculous, I mean this whole fucking thing is ridiculous. I just don't get me, I don't understand all of this. I get it but I don't fucking understand it. Maybe it's just a case of letting things take their course, managing this and seeing where it takes me. Previous works I've gotten out what's bothering me, backstories, planning and even swearing on celibacy. Aye that lasted long. See? I make these grand fucking plans and within a week or a month I'm breaking them. Do you know the best thing to do? See any plan that I say I'm going to do, ignore it because it's all just a pile of absolute fucking pish. I have the greatest of intentions but the worst will. See if I really wanted to and I mean REALLY wanted to I could give up alcohol but... I won't. Whatever I say I'm going to do is all spur of the moment, it's all fiction, and basically it's all fucking tosh. I wouldn't say I give up because that's dramatic but I am at a total loss as to who I am. I've completely lost my identity and I have completely lost my way. I'm lost, I am hopelessly lost in my life and I don't know where to go, who to turn to or what my next move is. I'm back sitting at the road with one million junctions, it's pitch black and I'm blindfolded, I have no clue what's the first step to take, what direction I'm going in or what direction I want to take. I can make the simplest thing complex, pretty ironic for a guy that prides himself on wanting the simple things. The weird thing about this whole fucking stramash is that it speaks to me about how I need a direction in life, that much I get and I appreciate it but what it doesn't do is tell me why the fuck I'm feeling like this, why am I stuck between happiness & suicide, thunder & sunshine, chalk & cheese, any sort of opposite combination you want to stick in here then stick it in. What does it matter? What does any of this matter? It won't go away, I don't know if I want it to go away, I don't know what to do and I don't know if I'll ever know what I want to do. I may be contemplating this in thirty years, I may be dead within two years. Do you know what? I…. just.. don't know. Just how much am I expected to bleed before the wound heals? How much further do I have to run before I can stop? Just how many walls am I going to have to blitz through before I can relax? I'm thinking back to this time last year. This time last year was by far the worst time I've ever had, I'd say that's fair considering all I went through. I went on a course of anti-depressants (which done nothing) and I stayed with my brother. He went to work and I was in the house, I didn't wash my face for forty-four days, I fought with myself day in and day out for months, I spent a lot of my time in silence staring out into nothing, I spent my days wandering from room-to-room, not doing anything, aimlessly killing time until bedtime so I could sleep, at least when I slept nothing could hurt me. I spent the best part of four months wondering if I was ever going to be myself again, I spent four long, hard months trapped between being on my own and leaving the house. Did any of my so called friends come to see me? Did they fuck, the people that told me that 'if I ever needed a chat' that they'd be there for me. The people that wished me well and said that 'a catch-up soon would be nice' didn't bother their arse. I made the effort, I went out once in Glasgow in November but it was me that made the effort, I dragged myself up and out, I put myself in a place where I hadn't been in a while, I put myself right smack bang around people, I put myself in Glasgow where there were a lot of people, not once did I feel comfortable but it was up to me to make the effort. I guess I just wasn't that important after all, I guess some people are just so full of shit that they say what you want to hear and then just forget all about you. I spent four of the longest months searching for something to grab on to and the only thing that I really ended up grabbing onto was an alcohol addiction and a desire to commit suicide. That's what my four months got me, that was the sum total of my time. I have never felt so confused, I've never had that much time to myself and I've never hated myself that much. That tearing between being on my own and going down to see my folks, the debating, the staring out the window, the wandering. The doubt, fear and self-loathing I endured was nothing short of torture, quite frankly I'm not sure how I managed four months. Ok so eventually I tried to tap out and quit, no wonder. By the end of things I was nothing but an alcoholic, alcohol had lost it's flavour as I got hammered every night. If it wasn't for my true friends & my family I wouldn't be here. That's why I fight, that's why when this gets me down I remind myself of just how much I have fought to get back up to where I am today. Yes this is a bad period but I've had worse, I've had sustained periods where I have been held prisoner in my own mind. This? This is nothing compared to what I went through but it doesn't make it any easier. I'm writing this for a reason, there is a point to this self-mutilation. If I lay everything out there it means I can't hide, I can't hide away from it and I can't run away from it. By being honest about suicide it means I'm one step closer to finding a way to deal with this and maybe that one step is one of ten thousand, it doesn't matter. Any step I and anyone that suffers from a mental health issue can take towards being a better person I'll take, I don't care if that one step is over broken glass whilst bare-footed I'll take it. Hell I'll crawl if it means collectively we can fight through this. With mental health issues like depression just making it through a day is an achievement, by me making it through to seven am and getting to bed is an achievement. If by helping people I've got to slice myself open I'll do it. I can do it and I'm used to doing it. I bleed every day and I'm not afraid to show that. I'm a good man with a lot to give but the question I constantly ask is... Will I get the time to give back and I think it's only fair to answer it with this... I don't know. I need to do something but what? Will volunteering to help people that struggle with mental health give me what I need to release myself from this or am I destined to never be freed from this. Am I going to spend the rest of my life searching for something that maybe just.. isn't there? This much is for sure, my journey hasn't been an easy one but one of the things giving me comfort is I'm still going, I'm still fighting and I'm still maintaining hope that someday I can one day break through these walls and leave them all broken behind me. Maybe one day this'll all make sense and I can manage it effectively. Maybe one day I can accept myself for who I am. My life has fantastic people in it and I am so grateful to have them in it but do I want them knowing I suffer? Well, yes if I'm suffering then they need to know, the mistake I made last year was not doing that.

They thought I was fine and I wasn't, I mean I REALLY wasn't. Would I say I'm fine just now? Well, no of course I'm not because of what's been written but if it comes time to ask for help, I'll do it. Make no mistake, if I'm going to bow out I want to do it after I have explored every single option, my folks raised no quitter, I am not a quitter, I'm a scrapper and a fighter. By bleeding myself out I'm proving that I'm strong, by ripping my wounds wide open for everyone to see shows that I'm fighting. I am fighting, we're all fighting this and hopefully we can beat this. I want to keep writing things like this because it shows there is still fight left within me. If I'm not doing anything then I've given up and the story is finished, my journey has ended. I don't want my journey to end just yet, I'm not ready but for any reason if it does I need to have it cleared up that I fought, I fought with every bit of my heart, body and soul. I am fighting with heart, body and soul. This may not make a lot of sense to people that don't suffer from mental health issues but believe me, that statement shows there's still fight in the tank, there's still a fight going on and there's commitment. It shows that although I've acknowledged that suicide doesn't scare me it's not an option I'm going to turn to easily, it's not something I'm going to turn to without taking every single step I can to beat this. I do want to beat this but... ... it's just so draining sometimes.

To be honest I am still contemplating going this alone. I got burned badly last year by people whom I thought were my friends, that took a lot of getting over and that's only something that I've recently managed to deal with, attempting suicide took one month to get over, being burned by people that I thought were there for me has taken a long time to heal. I value friends and I mean I value FRIENDS, true friends. The kind of friends that stepped up last year when they knew I was miles off, the type of friends that brought me back from the edge of a balcony, friends that are there for me in the good times and also are there for me during the bad times. I worship these people, I need these people and I love these people but after last year and what I'm feeling now, is it maybe time for me to go this alone? I feel.. ...I feel a sense of overwhelming detachment from them and I just don't feel the same. I will never forget what they done but things are changing inside my mind, I feel I've lost my connection with them so I think I've got a decision to make. I love them so much and I mean that, that's why I think I need to step away from them, I'm no longer the same to them, I feel it. I've tried to re-connect but let's face it, there comes a point in your life where you look at something and you're like... nope. I think that's where I am now, I've ran as far as I can with my friends and now it's time for me to deal with this on my own whatever that means. The hardest part of this is going to be having the conversations with them. I'm sure I'll miss the good times they share but also it makes sense for me to make this decision. I need to face this on my own, I need to deal with this on my own and eventually a road will open, the darkness will lift and I'll take whatever path shines brightest. Which one that'll be... Well.. I don't know.

December 2015

I don't even know the reason as to why I'm writing, honestly I don't. All I know is this grips me, leaves me, smothers me and then fucks me, it's like a never-ending cycle and I don't have the energy to make some bold, brave statement about how 'I'm going to beat this' or 'how I'm going to fight through it'. All I know is I'm sitting here, it's 7:29am on 13/12/2015, Christmas is already a bad time of the year for me and now depression has decided that this would be a great time to rock up, in fairness I should have expected it, infact I don't know why I didn't see this coming. What exactly am I hoping to achieve here? What is my ultimate aim by writing about it? My hatred of people is intensifying, my utter hatred of Christmas is ramping up and on top of all that my desire to be everywhere and nowhere has reached fever pitch. Do you know something, fuck the above when I've referenced kindness, people listen but they don't understand, I don't blame them, I can't but I wish just for once I wish this would leave me the fuck alone.

www.ingramcontent.com/pod-product-compliance
Lightning Source LLC
Chambersburg PA
CBHW051211170526
45166CB00005B/1845

* 9 7 8 1 5 2 2 7 3 5 9 5 3 *